Welcome

Welcome

Patterns of the Moral Life

Lois Shepherd and Margaret Mohrmann

BLOOMSBURY ACADEMIC
NEW YORK • LONDON • OXFORD • NEW DELHI • SYDNEY

BLOOMSBURY ACADEMIC
Bloomsbury Publishing Inc
1359 Broadway, New York, NY 10018, USA
50 Bedford Square, London, WC1B 3DP, UK
29 Earlsfort Terrace, Dublin 2, Ireland

BLOOMSBURY, BLOOMSBURY ACADEMIC and the Diana logo are trademarks of Bloomsbury Publishing Plc

First published in the United States of America 2026

Copyright © Lois Shepherd and Margaret Mohrmann, 2026

For legal purposes the Acknowledgments on p. 252 constitute an extension of this copyright page.

Cover design: Diana Nuhn
Cover image © iStock/ cienpies

All rights reserved. No part of this publication may be reproduced or transmitted in any form or by any means, electronic or mechanical, including photocopying, recording, or any information storage or retrieval system, without prior permission in writing from the publishers.

Bloomsbury Publishing Inc does not have any control over, or responsibility for, any third-party websites referred to or in this book. All internet addresses given in this book were correct at the time of going to press. The author and publisher regret any inconvenience caused if addresses have changed or sites have ceased to exist, but can accept no responsibility for any such changes.

Scripture quotations are from New Revised Standard Version Bible, copyright © 1989 National Council of the Churches of Christ in the United States of America. Used by permission. All rights reserved worldwide.

Poem reprinted from *Ask the Moon, Collected Poems of Dannie Abse* copyright © 2026 Parthian. Used by permission. All rights reserved."

I Got A Name, Words by Norman Gimbel, Music by Charles Fox. @1973 (Renewed) Warner-Tamerlane Publishing Corp. All Rights Reserved. Used by Permission of Alfred Music.

Library of Congress Cataloging-in-Publication Data

ISBN: HB: 979-8-8818-0871-6
PB: 979-8-8818-0872-3
ePDF: 979-8-7651-5056-6
eBook: 979-8-8818-0873-0

Typeset by Deanta Global Publishing Services, Chennai, India
Printed and bound in the United States of America

To find out more about our authors and books visit www.bloomsbury.com and sign up for our newsletters.

Contents

Introduction: Welcome to This Book   1

Part I What Welcome Is

1. Radical Openness   11
2. Responding Rather Than Reacting   17
3. Action   23
4. Step into the Room   31
5. Stay Awhile   37
6. Invite the Other Person In   45
7. Everyone Is at Home   51
8. Welcoming Ourselves   61

Part II Paying Attention

9. See a Human Being   67
10. See *This* Human Being   75
11. Who Is This Person *Right Now*?   81
12. Empathy Is Not Enough   89
13. Everything about a Person Matters   101

Part III Things We Can Do

14. Practice, Practice, Practice   109
15. Reconsider, Again and Again   119
16. Let People Tell You Who They Are   125
17. Pay Attention to Names   135
18. Come as You Are   143
19. Let Others Come as They Are   149
20. Check Your Agenda   153

21 Worry Less about Being Manipulated	157
22 Be Open to Interruptions	163
23 Put People before Principles	171
24 Help Others Welcome You	181

Part IV How Far Do We Have to Go?

25 Welcome Can Be Costly	189
26 Managing Aversions: No One Is Unworthy of Being Welcomed	199
27 Making Choices, Setting Limits	211
28 Sharing the Responsibility	221
29 A Fundamental View of the World	229
30 Step into the Welcoming World	239
Epilogue: Further Steps	243
Appendix	245
Acknowledgments	252
Index	255
Index of Stories	258

Introduction

Welcome to This Book

This book is about why and how welcome matters and about how we can become more welcoming people.

Being a welcoming person is not just one of many moral commitments. It is and must be the primary commitment of people who wish to lead ethical lives. We may think of welcome primarily as a quality incumbent upon people in certain roles or certain situations, but welcome is owed by *everyone* to *everyone* else. It is the responsibility of both teacher and student, cashier and customer, lawyer and client, bus driver and passenger, and so on, to welcome each other. In the context of healthcare delivery, for example, this means not only doctors and nurses should be welcoming (and welcomed) but housekeepers, security guards, administrators, patients and their families, and more. And, just as everybody matters, *everything* matters, including such apparently mundane issues as whether we make eye contact and remember someone's name. The moral life is not limited to negotiating occasional ethical dilemmas. Each encounter and action related to another person has ethical significance. The understanding of the obligation of welcome presented in this book thus applies to every encounter, *every time*: We are *always* called to be welcoming.

Only by welcoming each other—willing ourselves to be open and attentively responsive to each person (see Part I)—is it possible for us to fathom our *responsibility* in an actual situation, to see clearly to whom we are responsible and for what. This claim may seem to suggest that the primary focus is on responsibility, and there are, without doubt, multiple resonances and resemblances between responsibility and welcome in human ethical life. Being responsive and recognizing responsibility are crucial components of a fully welcoming disposition. In fact, this project originally had the working title "Welcoming Responsibility," with near-equal attention devoted to the two terms. However, as we explored the depths and nuances of what it means to be a welcoming person, we came to see that welcome is *prior*. Welcome and responsibility are closely connected, each informing and expanding the other, but welcome is the essential entry point into discerning responsibilities well and living a responsive and responsible life.

This book presents welcome in three of the ways in which ethics is generally understood. Welcome is a *character trait* (a virtue or settled disposition), a *perspective* from which to envision how we may live together well, and an *obligation* that spurs us to action. More, we believe welcome is the *primary* virtue, perspective, and obligation without which other important ethical ways of being, seeing, and doing cannot be effectively and consistently achieved. It is welcome's open, attentive presence with the other person that enables us to determine what further ethical thought or action is called for, where professional obligations come into play, what moral requirements are at stake in the moment, and how they may best be fulfilled. That is, welcome is the "first work"—and the sine qua non—of other ethical approaches. We cannot reason well ethically or act well morally if we have not *first* paid sufficient attention to the persons involved in the situation we are facing, including ourselves.

Welcome can also be seen as closely linked with love, especially as love is understood by traditions of thought that emphasize an obligation to love one another. But as all of us are likely to have experienced, it is often quite difficult to know what love calls us to *do* in particular circumstances. It can be distressingly easy to settle for simply having generally loving feelings. However, by being welcoming—radically open to the other person, as we explain and illustrate in Part I and throughout the book—we can discern the good to be done, the fitting actions that express love, and be moved to act. Here, too, welcome is the first work.

Relating welcome to love raises immediate questions about connections between this concept of welcome and religious ideas and beliefs. This is not a book about religion; it is a work in practical normative ethics, the branch of ethical inquiry that explores standards of right and wrong and asks how we should behave, morally speaking. It neither relies upon nor rejects religious faith or any of religion's many and varied traditional paths. For some readers, religious commitments may add depth or nuance to discussions they find here or provide motivation for the sort of attention and practice that welcome requires. Religious perspectives may challenge—and be challenged by—the ideas presented. We encourage this kind of thoughtful interplay.

In the numerous brief chapters that follow—we call them "patterns" (see below)—we show the nature and effects of welcome, and of its absence. To do this, we mostly employ stories with commentary rather than theoretical arguments.[1] We promote *perspectives* consistent with a welcoming orientation (Part II) and suggest *practices* that can help us become more welcoming (Part III), both by increasing our openness to others and by removing or setting aside the particular obstacles to welcome that we each carry with us (explored more in Part IV). Our exploration ranges from simple moves of courtesy—for example, using names well—to complex and costly interactions, such as welcoming a stranger who is also a murderer. And, though we focus mainly on one-on-one encounters for clarity, we show that groups of people, as communities and institutions, also have an obligation to be welcoming, and we suggest ways in which we can share those responsibilities and support each other, welcoming those who, in turn, welcome others.

Backstory

Every book has a backstory about why its authors chose their topic and what they bring to it. For both of us, Lois and Margaret, this work is based on our particular education and experience. It is the culmination of many years of teaching and collegial interactions in higher education, but also draws from our involvement in family life, community activities, and faith traditions.

Lois is a law professor with a particular interest in the ethics of biomedicine and health care. It was through immersion in the work of Emanuel Levinas (in a course taught by a friend that she joined almost by chance) that she recognized "welcome" as not only a concept that usefully interpreted and explained her understanding of human moral obligations but also as a practice that could result in a more deeply ethical clinical medicine, health policy, and even law.

Margaret is a (retired) pediatrician and professor of theological ethics and medical education. During her graduate work and subsequent teaching in religious studies, she became familiar with the work of scholars such as H. Richard Niebuhr and Margaret Urban Walker and found that their explications of responsibility provided a route to framing her professional experience and creating a meaningful approach to the moral formation of medical practitioners.

We came to the writing of this book drawn by the obvious importance, to ethics and to the moral life, of people's willingness to be open and attentive to each other—and found in *welcome* the language with which to examine and present our convictions. Each of us also came to the project full of stories, episodes experienced or heard about during the course of our work in healthcare and medical education, that seemed clearly to illustrate salient facets of welcome. Given the intimacy of the encounters and the weight of the responsibilities common in the medical setting, stories that arise there offer memorable instruction about the remarkably positive power of welcoming acts as well as the dauntingly negative effects of failures to welcome. Thus, we initially thought of the book as a contribution to medical ethics, with welcome being a concept captured minimally or not at all in standard discussions of healthcare ethics and education.

Over the fifteen years in which we developed and refined our ideas, our creative process entailed innumerable conversations in which we continually circled back to these narratives, finding more in them, letting them take us further into understanding the nature and effects of welcome. As a result of this method, we became increasingly certain that our underlying premise is broadly applicable, that welcome is indeed incumbent on everyone, at every time, and the moral implications of and need for a welcoming disposition reach well beyond the ethics of healthcare alone to include every sphere of human interaction. We found other relevant stories everywhere—in novels and newspapers, and in our encounters with family, friends, and strangers outside of work. Over time, the book became not primarily a project within medical ethics but a proposition about the moral life generally understood, about how we treat each other, interact with each other, live with each other, in every setting. Ethics is most basically defined as the area of human thought and teaching that deals with how we each live and how we live together (including how we live in relation to the world, animate and inanimate). This, then, is a book about ethics, an ethics of welcome—for everyone.

In what follows, somewhat over half of the stories we present are healthcare related in some fashion, and thus that field can be said to serve as the primary "demonstration project" through which we present our broader claims. But this book invites and encourages readers to think about and through the lens of their own experiences, stories from work, family life, community activities, the daily news that come to mind as they read. We have brought to this exploration of welcome the narratives with which we are familiar; please bring yours.

The Structure of the Book

This book offers not a linear argument that progresses from hypothesis to evidence to conclusion but rather numerous interrelating, interweaving examples of thought and behavior that do or do not serve human harmony and flourishing. Welcoming others is itself not a linear process but one that constantly circles back on itself, expanding, adjusting, changing, as the welcomer and the one welcomed continue to learn from and respond to each other—and the same is inevitably true about in-depth discussions of welcome.

We attempt to mirror that process, as far as possible, in the structure of this work and, therefore, the book is assorted into *patterns*. In this, we have been inspired and assisted by *A Pattern Language*, an iconic book on architecture published in 1977.[2] That work presents and explicates patterns of human thought and behavior fundamentally important for planning and constructing towns and buildings for a healthy, peaceful, and equitable society. Though in many ways these are very different projects, both books are about *liveability*, about paying careful attention to the details of how we live in order that we might thrive together. Following the model of *A Pattern Language*, each of our patterns begins with one or more declarative statements that assert something true about welcome and about human beings and how we flourish together. The text of the pattern, centered on one or more stories, draws out the implications of those claims, and the pattern ends with imperatives—what we can do—that arise from that discussion.

Together, the patterns form a circular or, perhaps better, spiraling thought experiment that reveals what our lives and our human community could be like if we were all more truly welcoming persons. Each pattern calls out and answers to other patterns; each is incomplete or not fully realized without the others, which, when read—or, better, put into practice and lived—deepen the understanding of what has been read or practiced before. There is always more to see and learn and do.

Because of this interplay among the patterns, it may be valuable for many readers to read through the book from start to finish and then come back to reread patterns near the beginning or ones that left them uncomfortable or puzzled. Aspects of all patterns, perhaps especially those first encountered, will be more fully realized when understood with the whole. On the other hand, others may prefer to select patterns to read in no particular order, aiming for those that catch their attention from the Table of Contents or a riffle through the pages or an exploration of the detailed index (which shows, among other things, where a story presented in one pattern appears in another pattern in support of a different point). Or a reader may want to revisit certain patterns after having been involved in a similar situation, now bringing their own experience to their understanding.

Another image—that of "argument as dance"—may be useful for grasping not only the nonlinear nature of the argument but also the way we intend to interact with other, related ethical claims. In *Metaphors We Live By*, George Lakoff and Mark Johnson, in demonstrating that metaphorical concepts structure our everyday activity, assert that we often consider and perform "argument as war." We engage in "verbal battle" and structure our arguments in the form of "attack, defense, counterattack."[3] Then they suggest an alternative:

> Imagine a culture where an argument is viewed as a dance, the participants are seen as performers, and the goal is to perform in a balanced and aesthetically pleasing way. In such a culture, people would view arguments differently, experience them differently, carry them out differently, and talk about them differently.

A fundamental assumption of this book is that human flourishing looks like open, inclusive, welcoming communities of persons who create and sustain those communities by paying careful, responsive attention to each other. We do not attempt to prove or defend that belief but rather "perform" our supposition that we and our societies thrive when welcoming people carry out welcoming acts. Throughout, we engage with other thinkers, ancient and modern, who also offer in-depth thinking about the nature of human flourishing and paths toward its achievement. We are moving with them—out there on the dance floor, trying to figure it out together—with the common purpose of understanding and fostering good human relations, the prospect that moves us all.

We have said that the book is about why and how welcome matters. In what follows, we focus primarily on *how* questions: How should one who wishes to be welcoming act in this situation? How am I to look at what's happening here and now? How does one become a welcoming person? It is our belief that studying the *how* of welcome and the ethical life it promotes reveals the *why*. The picture that develops in this book of what a world of welcome would look like is appealing enough—*humane* enough—to speak for itself as to the why of welcome.

And the project is not complete. We have spent years working out the concepts presented here but appreciate that our observations and conclusions are limited by our knowledge and experience and that the illustrations we have selected may not best capture the essence of a particular human need or desire or challenge. The "solutions" and suggestions we offer are attempts, after digging deeply, to formulate reasonable responses to the questions we raise, but they are sure to fall short in one way or another. Patterns of human interaction have been evolving for eons, and there is no reason to think that they are somehow completed by being captured in the snapshots we offer. Besides, they *cannot* be complete for individual readers. Readers bring their own knowledge and experiences to understanding what welcome requires, what it costs, what it achieves, how it rewards.

Come, dance with us toward a more welcoming world.

Notes

1 In each of the stories we use, we alter names and identifying details as needed to protect confidentiality.
2 Christopher Alexander, Sara Ishikawa, Murray Silverstein et al., *A Pattern Language: Towns, Buildings, Construction* (New York: Oxford University Press, 1977).
3 George Lakoff and Mark Johnson, *Metaphors We Live By* (Chicago: University of Chicago Press, 1980), 4–5.

Part I

What Welcome Is

The patterns in Part I cover what is meant by welcome and what an ethics of welcome asks of us in terms of preparation and action, which we describe as movement—being moved and moving. The external movement that welcome requires can overcome the distance between the welcomer and the one welcomed and create a shared space.

1

Radical Openness

Welcome is a radical openness to the other person that both allows us to be moved and compels us to move in order to create, repair, and maintain the shared space necessary for responsible human relationships.

A welcoming stance is an *open* stance—open to the ones we wish to welcome, as they are; open to ourselves, as we are; open to what may now be possible. It is a stance that enables, motivates, and guides our appropriately responsive actions toward and on behalf of those we welcome.

> A man named Don Ritchie lived with his wife Moya in a house just across the street from the leading suicide spot in Australia, a steep cliff that overlooks the entrance to Sydney Harbor. For over 50 years, Don Ritchie watched from his window. When he saw someone standing at the edge of the cliff, he hurried over, offered a warm smile, asked if they'd like to talk, and invited them for a cup of tea, back in the kitchen where Moya had put on the kettle. They are believed to have saved well over 500 lives.
>
> Ritchie, who came to be known as the "Australian Angel," said, "You can't just sit there and watch them. You gotta try and save them. It's pretty simple." Don and Moya said they believed the location of their home was a gift. They never considered moving away but lived there, watching by the window, until Don died in 2012 at the age of 85.[1]

In order to interact so powerfully with all the strangers whom they called away from the cliff, we believe the Ritchies must have intentionally taken a welcoming stance. This required them to make choices. Some of these choices were physical, action-oriented. They chose to stand or sit by the window and to look in the direction of the cliff. They chose to approach the stranger and then to invite them into their house. They smiled, they gestured, they made tea. They moved in ways that placed them closer to the stranger in distress, rather than farther away. There they were, year after year, stepping out toward person after person who came to that cliff.

These choices of physical placement and action were made following or in concert with a more fundamental, equally intentional movement: the opening of their minds, hearts, and spirits—names we give to the parts of ourselves that perceive and respond to others. Welcome is an emotional, cognitive, spiritual, physical opening and extending of ourselves toward the one we welcome. The physical movement may often be a literal reaching out or stepping forward, as the Ritchies did, although at times welcome's moves are more subtle (eye contact, for example) or may even be restrained, taking a step back in order to respect a boundary or gain a clearer perspective.

The Ritchies didn't move away. Rather, they *intended* to live in this way. Welcome is about intention, about choosing, willing to be a certain kind of person—a claim grounded in the etymology of the word "welcome."[2]

"Welcome" has its root in ancient Anglo-Saxon languages and, therefore, is directly related to the German *willkommen*, a connection which demonstrates that the basic meaning of the word includes the *will*. That is, when I welcome you, I'm not really saying "well come," it is well or good that you have come. That's a related idea and a fine one: to see someone's coming as a good thing is surely a good thing. But the "wel" part of "welcome" does not mean "well"; it means "will." When I welcome you, I am affirming that your coming is in accord with my *will*: I will it. I want, I desire, I intend, I choose that you are here, that you have come here now. Put succinctly, "I welcome you" means "I want you to be here." It is about my intentions and my choices.[3]

"I welcome you" means "I want you to be here." It's not just "Okay, I accept that you're here. You're the next person in line for me to counsel or serve soup to, so come on in." A welcoming orientation means that my will, my intention is engaged: I *want* this, I want to encounter *you*, I want you to be in my presence, and I want to be in yours. I weave you into my life today.

The presence of this particular individual—*this* person, with their own stories, behaviors, beliefs, appearance—is wanted, and the person is welcomed as a unique human being, not as a type of human being, like "the elderly" or "diabetics" or "the homeless." Even if the person has behaviors or attributes that we don't like, the person is valued and welcomed as she is, as he is, as they are. Welcome says "Come as you are" and means it.[4]

Throughout the book, we explain welcome primarily in terms of one-on-one interactions, an approach that lends lucidity and simplicity to our presentations of various perspectives and practices. But, clearly, welcoming others is not always just a matter of individuals encountering each other. At various points, especially in Patterns 28 and 29, we explore welcome in the context of larger groups of people, focusing on the influence of a welcoming orientation (or its absence) on judicial decisions, community attitudes, and institutional policies. Even when we consider welcome as an obligation for a manufacturing business, a panel of judges, a refugee resettlement organization, a neighborhood, or a hospital, we are still talking about persons making decisions and undertaking actions that affect other persons.

The story of the Ritchies may call to mind another story, that of the "Good Samaritan." Originating in Christian scripture, the tale so resonates with human aspirations that it has often been used to illustrate secular discussions of our ethical obligations to each other, in healthcare and elsewhere. This story and the particular way it is told in its earliest versions offer further understanding of welcome and the central importance and interrelation of intention and movement, being moved by and moving toward another.

> "A man was going down from Jerusalem to Jericho and fell into the hands of robbers, who stripped him, beat him, and went away, leaving him half dead." Twice someone came by and saw the man, but continued on without stopping. Then a Samaritan man came near, "and when he saw him, he was moved with pity." The Samaritan dressed his wounds, took him to a nearby inn, and paid for his care there.[5]

Each of the three travelers who came down the road saw the injured man. What distinguishes the Samaritan is that he saw *and was moved*. The word translated here as "moved [with pity]" denotes, both in the original Greek and in the later Latin version, a visceral change, a deep internal shift in the Samaritan. The Latin word is *misericordia*. Usually translated as mercy or compassion, *misericordia* literally means that the Samaritan's heart (*cordia*) was twisted, wrung (*miser*). Today we might say his heart was wrenched or even broken by what he saw. *Misericordia* also aptly describes the Ritchies, moved by and toward what they saw.

How is it that some people are moved by persons and situations they encounter, and some are not? It is a matter of the will: the *intention* to live the kind of life in which one is aware of and responsive to others. It is this determined intention, reinforced by preparation and practice, that enables us to become persons who are *open* to being affected, moved by those we meet, and thus to become truly welcoming persons.

The Ritchies and the Samaritan were in some way prepared; they were *ready* not only to see the persons who appeared in their lives but to be moved by them and to respond to them accordingly. Some interpreters of the Samaritan story have claimed that the Samaritan must have been a physician to explain why he stopped—an odd and unsupported interpolation into the tale. Even if the Samaritan were someone trained in the healing arts, that doesn't explain his response. We know by experience that we cannot assume that a person is sure to be moved by the plight of another simply by virtue of having an MD degree or, for that matter, an RN, MSW, MDiv, or any other credential that allows entry into a healing, caring profession. Don Ritchie was an insurance salesman. Whatever the day jobs held by our exemplars, whatever they were educated or trained to do, all we can say for certain, on the information given, is that they were open, available, and responsive: open to seeing the injured man on the road and the hurting people who came to the cliff as they were; open to being drawn toward them, to being moved to approach, to see and hear more.

That *openness*—the disposition to see, to perceive, and to respond—is a particular way of being in the world: the habit or disposition or virtue of *welcome*, of being a welcoming person. Our exemplars acted the way they did because, *first*, they were open, ready and willing to welcome into their minds and their hearts the persons who came into view.

When we intend to be open to others—aware of who they are, what they've experienced, what they may need—we are at the same time choosing to be responsive to what we perceive and learn. That is, welcome is not, cannot be, a passive, purely receptive phenomenon. The internal movements—the wrenching of the heart, illumination of the mind, disturbance of the spirit that inevitably arise from being open and available to those we encounter—compel action, external movements that respond appropriately to what we are now aware of (see Patterns 2 and 3). The responding action may be as subtle as a nod of acknowledgment, as dramatic as a full-fledged, perilous rescue, or anything in between those extremes, but it is *action*. The Ritchies stepped out on the cliff and invited the stranger in for tea; the Samaritan knelt beside the injured man and carried him to safety.

Note, too, that welcome is the obligation we have toward persons who appear before us—the spouse across our breakfast table, the client in our office, our fellow classmates, our tired boss, the stranger sitting next to us at the meeting, the clerk bagging our groceries, the person we stumble over or glimpse through our window who is in obvious need of help. That is, the obligation of welcome does not require us to seek out persons to welcome; it does not ask that we all become beaming extroverts, rushing up to the new person in the room. The primary movement of welcome is not thrusting ourselves toward someone but opening ourselves to them (see Pattern 7).

We have written this book with the assumption that anyone who reads it is interested in being, or becoming, a welcoming person. That intention, even if only nascent, is the necessary first step to becoming open to the reality of other persons, available to be moved by them, able to move toward them in responsive and responsible ways. Much of the book, then, explores what such openness entails (including the potential costs and perils), how we can become more thoughtfully and deliberately open, and what the results of such a stance may be.

Open yourself to others as they are. Allow yourself to be moved by them.

Notes

1. "Australian 'Angel' Saves Lives at Suicide Spot," *CBS News*, June 14, 2010. https://www.cbsnews.com/news/australian-angel-saves-lives-at-suicide-spot/.
2. Explorations of etymology can uncover depths of meaning. As Daniel Mendelssohn wrote about the provenance of words, "the places they come from . . . can tell us something about what we've thought, over the centuries and millennia, about just what this act consists of and what it means" (Daniel Mendelssohn, *An Odyssey: A Father, A Son, and An Epic* [Knopf, New York, 2017], 20).
3. Another etymological point: "Welcome" does not have a Latin root. Words for "welcome" in Romance languages—such as *bienvenue* in French, *bienvenido* in Spanish—do mean "well come," but they are direct borrowings from what the English word "welcome" *sounds* like; they don't have Latin roots of their own. That said, there is a Latin word that denotes the understanding of "welcome" that permeates this book: *complecto*. This verb, in addition to expressing "welcome," also means "embrace, encircle, encompass." Composed of the prefix *com-* (with, together) and the verb *plecto* (to plait or braid, to weave), the Latin version of "welcome" contains the rich metaphor of weaving together, of welcome as an entwining embrace, joining us in one fabric, a shared relational space.
4. No doubt, the word "welcome" can be used—misused—in ways antithetical to its meaning. We may say, sarcastically, "Welcome to my world," or, with malice, "Welcome to the worst day of your life." The sentiment expressed in such statements is obviously *not* a welcoming one, and the intended meaning should not be taken seriously as a construal of the concept of welcome.
5. Quoted parts are from the story as recounted in the New Testament (NRSV) in Lk. 10:25-37.

2

Responding Rather Than Reacting

Welcome is not a reaction but a response *to the particular person before us.*

Consider this "case summary" presented to one of us several years ago for commentary:

> JR is an 84-year-old man with moderate dementia and significant heart disease who has an aggressive renal tumor.

Were we to give this one-sentence sketch to a group of health practitioners or medical ethicists, some, perhaps many, would confidently declare that the right thing to do is not to operate on JR's tumor. Surgical intervention would be too risky, too likely to add to his suffering, too unlikely to change his future significantly. Rather, they might say, the right thing to do is provide compassionate palliative care so he will be comfortable until the tumor or the dementia or the heart disease ends his life. Whether these opinions are "correct" or not is arguable, but what is not debatable is that they are, and can only be, a *reaction* to the bare information given. They are not a *response* to "JR" the person because he remains unknown to the commentators.

When we welcome someone, we do not simply offer a reply—a yes/no/maybe answer—to their questions or requests nor do we just react to them, triggered by some attribute or initial impression. In welcoming another, we *respond* to them. Openness (Pattern 1) and responsiveness are closely linked, even inseparable, components of welcome. Together they are the clearest expression of welcome's defining declaration: "I want you here." Openness to another person moves us to respond and enables us to discern what responses may be appropriate.

H. Richard Niebuhr, an influential mid-twentieth-century theological ethicist, was one of the early proponents of "responsibility ethics," an understanding of the moral life that puts the ability to be responsive at the center of human community and of all our activities together—teaching, learning, parenting, playing basketball, healthcare, selling, banking, everything. Niebuhr argued that we are always in a stance of response, always responding to someone or to some state of affairs. Responsibility is the center of what we do and of who we are, and our moral goodness depends on how well we do it. He said that our primary moral task, then, is to discern the response that is most appropriate to the situation at hand, to find the *fitting* thing to do or to say.[1]

What would it take to move from reaction to the "case" of JR toward a fitting response to the person JR? We must start by asking, Who is JR? The use of initials to identify someone who is the subject of a case discussion is a long-standing tradition in medical case presentations, intended to protect the patient's privacy. Initials, however, are a thin veil, like the ineffective "privacy curtains" in shared hospital rooms. Worse, the use of initials is literally and quite effectively dehumanizing. "JR" becomes Everyman—and, thus, no one—as his own particularity is lost along with his name (see Pattern 17).

We'll give JR a name—invented for this discussion—in an effort to recover and foreground the person whose life and well-being are at stake in the decisions being considered, the person to whom we must be responsive and responsible. We'll call him John Rembert. All the details in the JR case sketch—dementia, heart disease, tumor—are still true, but they are not all that's true and relevant about John Rembert. The physician who initially presented the case added a few details that help fill out the picture a bit. Mr. Rembert is a fisherman who has spent his life on the water and, even in his eighties, despite increasing cognitive and physical difficulty, still enjoys being on the water and helping with the shellfish harvest. Mr. Rembert is also Uncle John, part of a family that includes a niece who looks out for him, accompanies him to see the doctor, and carries his medical and financial power of attorney.

There's more we could say about John Rembert, if we only knew it. Maybe he's good ol' John, beloved friend to many, especially his fellow watermen, the ones he's worked with for more than sixty years. Maybe he's Elder Rembert, pillar of his church community. Maybe he's Johnny the hell-raiser whose neighbors wonder how he's managed to survive this long. Maybe he's all of these things, maybe not, but he is certainly more than an age and a handful of diagnoses. Moreover, whatever the extent of his dementia, there is likely to be much we can learn directly from him. What does he want? What does he care about? It is John Rembert the whole person who requires our response, and everything knowable about him has a role in shaping a response that is appropriate.

Of course, with further clarity about who John Rembert is, the simplicity achieved by distilling the "case" into one sentence will undoubtedly be lost. We may fear that knowing more about someone just complicates things and makes us less able to step forward on their behalf—as we must in certain situations, medical and otherwise—because we may be stymied by the incorrigible ambiguities inherent in real human lives as well as in professional knowledge. However, there is no way around the fact that the *less* we know about someone else, the more likely we are to miss the mark, to be flat-out wrong, and even harmful in our deliberations and interactions.

Throughout this book, there are numerous stories that demonstrate the many ways in which a good intention to welcome someone can be derailed by our reacting instead of responding to them. What distinguishes a response from a reaction?

In Amor Towles' 2016 novel, *A Gentleman in Moscow*, Count Rostov (the main character) meets a well-known actress who will become a very important person in his life. At that first meeting, he forms certain quick judgments about her, based largely on his interpretation of her self-presentation and his awareness of her celebrity. But his initial negative, dismissive reaction—his "first impression"—is quickly overturned when they share a meal together and he begins to know her. The Count muses on this experience:

> After all, what can a first impression tell us about someone we've just met for a minute in the lobby of a hotel? For that matter, what can a first impression tell us about anyone? Why, no more than a chord can tell us about Beethoven, or a brushstroke about Botticelli. By their very nature, human beings are

so capricious, so complex, so delightfully contradictory, that they deserve not only our consideration but our *reconsideration*—and our unwavering determination to withhold our opinion until we have engaged with them in every possible setting at every possible hour.[2]

Our reactions to persons we encounter tend to arise from something within *us*—associative memories, habitual stances, fears, needs—sparked by our immediate interpretation of the person, our first impression. But that construal may have little to do with the full reality of the other person, yet to be recognized and acknowledged. Thus, reactions are not likely to be acts of welcome.

Reactions are reflexes and, as such, they are hasty and unthinking, impulsive, inattentive, involuntary—and generic, only loosely connected to the actual person to whom we are reacting. In contrast, responses are deliberate and thoughtful, reflective, attentive, chosen, and specific to the person and the circumstances.[3]

In the context of John Rembert's situation, given the "case" summary, a medical ethicist may think reflexively of past similar cases and discussions, a surgeon or a nurse immediately recall past experiences with similar patients and the emotions connected to them. It is not that these reactive considerations are useless or irrelevant; it is that they are not enough and may even stand in the way of good reasoning on behalf of this particular person. Further acquaintance with John Rembert and his life won't magically reveal a singular correct answer to the question of whether to remove his renal tumor, but it will make it significantly more likely that the decision reached is responsive and responsible, fits who he is, what he wants, how he lives, what he values.

This claim is not an argument against case-based ethical deliberation. A thought experiment about an abstracted "case" can be instructive and, at times, helpful for moving beyond reflex reactions. However, whatever may be gleaned from reasoning about JR, our primary moral engagement is always with John Rembert. It is the particular details of his existence, in all their complexity, and of his desires, difficult as they may be to discern, that determine whether our responses to him and to his situation are fitting.

It is also important to note that responses not only must fit the person being welcomed and the particularities of the situation, but also must fit the welcomer, the one responding. The decisions made by John Rembert's physician and by his niece should be, as far as possible, in line with—and certainly should not violate—their understandings of their responsibilities and commitments. At the same time that we welcome others, we are always also welcoming ourselves (see Pattern 8), and the crucial call for a fitting response applies to everyone in the encounter.

"Ability to respond" is the core meaning of "responsibility." This is surely an obvious claim, but we often forget this basic definition as we juggle all the various "responsibilities" in our lives and use the word as nothing more than a synonym for "task" or "obligation." In this discussion of the essential elements of welcome, however, responsibility is not a task but a character trait, the attribute of consistently *being a responsible person*, one who can and does respond, rather than react, to a person one encounters.

If we wish to be welcoming, we must be responsible. Conversely, if we want to be responsible persons, we have to be welcoming persons as well, willing to invest the attention to others necessary for our responses to be more and other than merely answers that stop the questions or reactions that impede the flow of communication and the growth of relationship.

It may not be possible, or even always desirable, to prevent spontaneous first impressions from arising when we meet someone for the first time or when we encounter someone we know well in a new situation. However, we can notice those reactions and set them aside in order to give our full attention to the whole person before us, seeking to know what we must in order to respond in ways that fit the one we welcome and the relationship between us.

Learn to recognize reactions for what they are. Choose instead to respond.

Notes

1   H. Richard Niebuhr, *The Responsible Self: An Essay in Christian Moral Philosophy* (New York: Harper & Row, 1963), 47–68 *et passim*.

2 Amor Towles, *A Gentleman in Moscow* (New York: Viking, 2016), 120–1.
3 This distinction between a reaction and a response is supported by the observation that the Latin *responsus*, the direct ancestor of "response," denotes harmonious agreement or "correspondence" with someone. Its root is in the verb *spondeo*, which means to promise, take a sacred vow, or contract in marriage, as can be seen in other English words that arose from it, such as "sponsor" and "spouse." The addition of the prefix *re-* introduces a sense of reverberation, a sustained movement back and forth between two or more mutually responsive actors.

3

Action

Welcome is openness and responsive action.

Welcome requires emotional, spiritual, cognitive, and physical movement. The requirement of physical movement, of some physical act that we undertake, is part of what distinguishes an ethics of welcome from conventional understandings of love or compassion or empathy (see also Pattern 12). Here, we discuss the relationship between *being moved*—the internal stirrings of welcome, of responsive openness—and *moving*, the external actions thus compelled.

> A medical student spoke of a patient to whom he was assigned: At the time the patient was admitted, there had been hope for recovery of at least some level of good function, but since then things had gone downhill. The patient was now lying in an intensive care unit and would die there. She continued to have some awareness of her surroundings, but "there was nothing more the doctors could do for her," the student said. He now found himself avoiding going into her room, walking straight by it, because he believed he had nothing to offer. He felt terrible for her. But, he explained, he also just felt terrible, period.

Congruence between our internal stirrings and external actions is a significant component of individual integrity. It is also crucial for being a welcoming person. Welcome depends upon our being affected in some way—moved—by the one to whom we open ourselves, but it also requires that we act in fitting response to that visceral shift. In the fullness of welcome, internal movements must lead to welcoming action, some sort of movement, simple or complex, toward the other person. Empathy—"feeling terrible" for or with someone— is never enough by itself. Imagine if the Ritchies, those Australian Angels introduced in the first pattern, noticing someone outside their window poised to jump from the cliff, had said to each other, "Such a pity," and then with moist eyes turned back to watch the television news.

Welcome entails both being moved *and* moving in response to that stimulus to in some way acknowledge, support, accompany, assist, or otherwise embrace the one who has moved us, the one we want to welcome. The medical student in the story above experiences disturbing feelings about the patient he was avoiding, but he takes no steps toward her. If we accept his self-description that he is indeed moved by her plight, we can speculate that his inability to move toward her may be a matter of inexperience and fear—each of which can eventually be remedied by teaching, modeling, encouragement, and practice.

Contrast the medical student's account with the following. This story, too, is about a patient experiencing a terminal condition for whom medicine had nothing to offer in the way of a cure.

> Mark Horowitz suffered quietly for years from both heart disease and chronic leukemia. In the months before his death, he often spoke of his encounter with a resident physician (a doctor in training). Mark had been admitted to the hospital because of a recurrence of his leukemia; he was quite sick and facing the likelihood that this was the beginning of the end for him, as it turned out to be. He had been poked and imaged and biopsied for hours that day in the clinic and now was relieved to be in his bed, in his quiet hospital room, finally alone with his thoughts. Then the resident came in. Mark, always a kind, welcoming man, would surely have smiled at him, but he wasn't particularly interested in telling his long medical story yet again.
>
> But then, to put it in Mark's words, "The resident just came in, sat down, looked at me, and said, 'Mr. Horowitz, how can I help you?'" This is the point at which Mark would start to cry, every time he told the story. Once he composed himself, he would explain that this was the most comforting, most embracing question he'd heard all day (and, he sometimes added, maybe through the entire course of his illnesses). He had not yet said one word to the resident, but he already felt heard and known and held.

Like the medical student who avoided the room of a dying patient, the resident also appears to have experienced empathy for his patient. But he responded differently; he *acted*. He entered the room, sat down, and stayed. The contrast is stark: the image of a closed door with someone walking by versus the image of an opened door with someone sitting beside the other person.

An ethics of welcome is not limited to the realm of healthcare, and it is also not solely about one-on-one meetings between two persons (see the discussion in Pattern 1, further developed in Patterns 28 and 29). It has something meaningful to say about the many ways in which we touch one another's lives—the lives of people we know and the lives of strangers—in an infinite variety of circumstances, including indirectly through institutional policies, laws, and court decisions.

> The United States Supreme Court case of *DeShaney v. Winnebago County Department of Social Services*[1] from 1989 was about a little boy, Joshua DeShaney, whose father beat him nearly to death. Joshua survived but was left with devastating brain injuries. A lawsuit brought on his behalf claimed that the state agency charged with protecting vulnerable people like Joshua had failed to protect him, that despite receiving reports of prior abuse the agency's staff had grossly neglected their duties to follow up and take protective measures on the boy's behalf.
>
> When the Supreme Court heard this case, they determined that Joshua had no right to protection from the state agency. Our Constitution protects only negative rights, the Court explained, rights to be free from governmental intrusions rather than rights to receive governmental protection. The Court made clear that no matter how egregious the decisions or actions of the state agency—whether callous, reckless, inept, or the blind result of bureaucratic arbitrariness (simply "because his name began with a J," as memorably noted by dissenting Justice Brennan)—the agency could not be sued and their actions would not be scrutinized. The majority opinion of the Court said that this conclusion was dictated by precedent, past cases. Nothing they could do.
>
> Yet the justices were careful to convey their compassion: "The facts of this case are undeniably tragic," they wrote. "Judges and lawyers, like other humans, are moved by natural sympathy in a case like this."

The Justices in the majority presented themselves as sympathetic, although they also distanced themselves from that claim, couching it in the third person (not "We are moved," but "[j]udges and lawyers, like other humans, are moved").[2] However, even if they were truly moved by Joshua DeShaney and what had happened to him, that internal effect did not in fact compel them to act responsively by allowing a full consideration of the facts and deliberating about whether they should create new precedent. Instead, they "retreated," to use Justice Brennan's words, "into a sterile formalism." The Court's majority opinion ticks through relevant prior cases and concludes, "But these cases afford petitioners no help," again choosing third-person language[3] to deny the Justices' own role in the decision to do nothing to help Joshua or others like him.

In this sense, the Supreme Court Justices who decided this case are similar to the medical student who expressed compassionate feelings toward his patient but walked by her room without entering it. Like the student (although lacking the student's excuse of inexperience), they needed to do the equivalent of entering Joshua's room—by attending to and being present with the particular facts of the particular case that bears his particular name—in order to welcome him into their courtroom and recognize their responsibility to him and others.

Earlier in this pattern, we point out that congruity between our internal stirrings and our external actions is necessary for personal integrity. Emmanuel Levinas—a philosopher whose writings deeply inform our discussion of welcome—went further. According to Levinas, *it is our response to the call of the other person that makes us human*. We exist as human beings, in effect, *only* because of other people and our responses to them. David Kangas, a professor of the philosophy of religion, described the phenomenon via the metaphor of a ringing telephone: If you answer the phone, you are there; if you do not, you are not. If you just let it ring and ring and ring, you are, in every way, "not there" for the person calling. You do not, or may as well not, exist.[4]

Joshua DeShaney called out for help all the way to the Supreme Court, but when his call arrived, it went unanswered. The Justices were not there; the place was empty.

The medical student described at the beginning of this pattern heard, in essence, a call ringing again and again as he passed the patient's room, but he did not answer. That's surely part of why he felt terrible, for each time his integrity and even his very humanness were called into question. By not answering the call, he simply wasn't there, did not exist for that person. The resident who attended to Mark Horowitz, in contrast, reaffirmed his own humanity along with that of his patient when he entered the room, sat down, and opened himself to the call.

For both the medical student and the Justices in the majority, action seems to have been stymied by, among other things, the actors' *confusion about their roles*. They have forgotten or set aside or do not know that the *first* and essential role for each of us is being a person in relation with other persons. Only then are our responses inflected by the more specific, individual roles we are in. No one—not doctors, judges, or anyone else—gets to skip that basic component of being human, part of the human community.

Further, the student and the Justices are hindered by their assumption that there is *nothing they can do*, whether to save a dying patient, undo damage already done, or overturn precedent. But the call to welcome others insists that we re-examine that claim whenever it arises. It certainly surfaces frequently in medical practice and regrettably often in political discourse, and it is always incorrect. Persons who are welcoming recognize that there is *always* something we can do, for they do not discount the real significance of the actions of welcome.

More experienced doctors can tell the student that he can indeed go into the patient's room to be with her, just as the resident could be present for Mark Horowitz even when there may have been "nothing to be done" about his illness. Similarly, Justice Brennan, in disagreeing with the majority's claim in the *DeShaney* case that the Court had no power to act, pointed out that the Court is, after all, the ultimate interpreter of the Constitution. It created the precedent and decided the past cases that it now claims tie its hands—and therefore, in fact, it does have the power to decide differently, to act in response to Joshua and his situation.

Both the student and the Justices asserted they were moved by the plight of a person they did not actually move toward. We have noted that the distancing language used by the Court majority calls the sincerity of its claim into question. We may also wonder if the student's feeling "terrible" could instead have been evoked by something other than his patient's condition—perhaps his concerns about the realities of the vocation he is training for or his fitness for it. That is, what if neither story is about someone moved but failing to act, but is instead about someone who was not, or not sufficiently, moved in the first place? How might such a situation—when internal stirrings are absent or dim—be remedied by one who truly wants to be welcoming? By action: We can move closer to and focus our attention on the one we want to welcome so that we may then be affected by them and their circumstances, interrupted, changed into someone who can and will respond fittingly.

The student may need to be encouraged to enter the patient's room and sit with her awhile, pay attention to her, allow the internal shift, the movement of heart and mind, to happen, and then let that experience instruct and motivate him to respond accordingly. Appellate courts deal in legal briefs and lawyers' presentations rather than hearing directly from plaintiffs and witnesses, but the Justices may have needed to do the equivalent of placing themselves in the presence of the petitioner Joshua DeShaney. That is, they could have paid careful attention to the story of how things unfolded for him, allowed themselves to be moved personally, not abstractly, their hearts to be wrenched (*misericordia*) by the realities of his current existence, and then let that experience help them to reconsider, to think again about what judicial responses may be possible and appropriate.

This is an example of the nonlinearity of the process of welcoming someone, as mentioned in our Introduction. In these first few patterns, we may seem to be setting out a simple progression of steps in welcome: I open myself to the other person, I am moved by that person, I respond with appropriate actions. Many times, the process of welcoming does flow from A to B to C, even smoothly enough that we don't notice the transitions. But it can also be the case that A, B, and C interact in different sequences. In order to open myself to someone in welcome, I may first have to make external movements, taking steps to come closer in order to be affected by them and discern what further measures would fit our circumstances. Those resulting actions, in turn, may allow me to see my partner in welcome more clearly or from another angle, influencing the next steps, and so on. What is consistent throughout is the need for overcoming distance, for *proximity*, physical or otherwise, as we discuss in the next pattern.

We cannot know if the Ritchies, the Australian Angels, were so moved by the mere sight of someone standing at the cliff that they felt compelled to reach out, or whether—at least the first or second time it happened—they chose to approach out of a sense of duty or horror and *then* found themselves profoundly moved by the persons they stood beside and invited into their home. The medical student, whether he is truly moved or has yet to allow that, must place himself in the presence of the patient to whom he has been assigned in order to welcome her as she is. And the Supreme Court Justices, rather than determining at the outset that the facts didn't matter, should have listened to and struggled with Joshua DeShaney's story.

Openness to others—our willed availability to being moved by them—is not static but active and responsive. Our ensuing actions may not make a severely injured child whole again or keep a patient from dying, but such outcomes, desirable as they may be, are not the only or even the most important reasons to be welcoming. Rather, fitting actions ensure that the one welcomed has been truly attended to, heard and known, held within the human community as a fully human being who is seen, acknowledged, and wanted.

The Supreme Court Justices in the majority would not have reversed Joshua DeShaney's brain injuries by opening themselves to the facts of his case and allowing themselves to be affected by them. But they could have recognized the urgency of the situation sufficiently to question a precedent and a construal of rights that left them unable to protect other children from suffering Joshua's fate by insisting that responsible agencies fulfill their responsibilities.

The medical student's patient, by all evidence available, would not have been saved from death by his entering the room and staying with her for a while. But, if she still had some level of awareness, she could have experienced the caring, attentive presence of another person there for her. And the student, if he opened himself to her, could have learned valuable lessons about doctoring and the power of presence, and perhaps even experienced some easing of his "terrible" feelings in that shared space that welcome creates.

The resident who cared for Mark Horowitz was both ready and willing to enter the patient's room and stay. He, too, could not save his dying patient, but he could and did offer comfort and understanding by his actions and by his simple, welcoming question, "How can I help you?"

Move!—in response to internal stirrings engendered by another person or in order to be so affected by them. Act!—responsively and responsibly.

Notes

1 *DeShaney v. Winnebago County Dep't of Soc. Servs.*, 489 U.S. 189 (1989).
2 Benjamin Zipursky, Note, "DeShaney and the Jurisprudence of Compassion," *New York University Law Review* 65 (1990): 1101.
3 Zipursky, "DeShaney," 1118.
4 Ethicist Laurie Zoloth, using Levinas' language to shift the focus of bioethics away from individual dignity and toward hospitality to the other, writes: "We are pulled toward the other in her complete need not because she is a pathetic victim but because *her interruption defines and authorizes our being.* Our abundant capacity for response is created by the way we must come up with what she needs even in a situation of scarcity" (emphasis added). Laurie Zoloth, "I Want You: Notes Toward a Theory of Hospitality," in *The Ethics of Bioethics: Mapping the Moral Landscape*, ed. Lisa A. Eckenwiler and Felicia Cohn (Johns Hopkins University Press, Baltimore, 2007), 205–19, at 210.

4

Step into the Room

Welcome is a physical act that overcomes the distance between persons.

Welcome says, "You are a person of value to me, and I desire to understand, know, and be with you." *I want to be with you.* Welcoming persons express that desire by moving toward the ones to be welcomed, overcoming the distance between them. Responsive movement in welcoming draws the welcomer closer to the other person emotionally, attentively, cognitively, and sometimes bodily. Welcome requires and seeks *proximity*, an immediacy that fosters relationship.[1]

What does proximity to the other person mean? What does it look like? What does it make possible?

Margaret tells of an experience from her residency in pediatrics. She is the "I" in the following story:

> One of my patients was a 12-year-old girl, Mickey, who had acute myelocytic leukemia. She was diagnosed in May, near the end of my internship year, and died in November of the same year. Mickey's last few weeks were spent in the Pediatric Intensive Care Unit (PICU), where she floated in and out of consciousness. Mary, her mother, spent those days sitting by her bedside. I popped in a few times each day, very aware that there was nothing that would prevent Mickey from dying, but not really knowing how to help her or her parents, or myself, get through the waiting time.
>
> After Mickey's death, I continued to spend time with her family. On one of my visits with them, Mary and I talked about how helpful the social worker, Ruth, had been throughout Mickey's illness. Mary started smiling, even chuckled a little, and then for the first time brought up those long, terrible days of Mickey's dying—and told me something I had not been aware of at the time: Every day they were in the PICU, Ruth came to the room and sat with them for close to an hour. Mostly they sat in silence,

but every fifteen minutes or so Ruth would look up, shake her head, and murmur "I don't know." Then silence again.

As Mary told me this story, she kept smiling, broadly—the only smile I ever saw from her when she talked about Mickey's dying. She offered no interpretation of what was happening in that room with Ruth, but she remembered it very clearly, and it made her smile.[2]

In the previous pattern, we relate the story of a medical student who avoided the room of a dying patient. Ruth did the opposite, day after day. She sat with Mickey and Mary. She voiced her and Mary's lack of comprehension and then also stayed silent, holding together with Mary their shared grief and pain in a sacred space of honesty, suffering, and responsiveness.

In order to form and flourish, relationships require that we be near to, in proximity with, the other person. The one who welcomes, the one who wills the other's presence, takes the steps necessary to get closer. Does it always have to be a physical closeness? No, it does not—but overcoming the distance between us and someone else is, nevertheless, always a physical act. As we explain in Pattern 3, the welcomer has to *do* something. Internal thoughts of welcome, feelings of openness to another person, stirrings of empathy are not enough.

Just as with writing: Lois' spouse, Paul Shepherd, explains to his writing students that writing is a physical activity. "How will I know if you're writing?" he asks them when it comes time for in-class writing. "Your fingers will be moving." The essay or novel or thank-you note in your head doesn't get written until there is physical movement, whether it's pen to paper, fingers to keyboard, dictation to a scribe, or even the blink of an eyelid. The latter is the means by which Jean-Dominique Bauby wrote the incomparable *The Diving Bell and the Butterfly* from his bed following a catastrophic stroke, signaling each chosen letter by blinking his left eyelid—the only part of him he could move—as an assistant ran her finger along the alphabet posted on a wall adjacent to his bed.

In several patterns in this book, we allude to the importance of understanding ourselves and others as whole persons, not separable into "parts" like body, mind, and spirit, and this is one example of that concept. There is no such thing as purely cognitive or purely spiritual expression; the body is always and essentially involved. How will it be evident that you've felt empathy for someone, been moved by them? You will be moving toward them in some way. You will be moving to overcome distance.

We say "overcome distance" rather than "reduce distance" in order not to unintentionally suggest that the distances are physical and that welcome requires us to place our body closer to the body of the one we welcome. Sometimes, obviously, it does, as the stories of the medical student and of the resident caring for Mark Horowitz in Pattern 3 and this pattern's story of Ruth sitting by Mickey's bedside illustrate. Sometimes, however, it is necessary to be less physically close to the other person, to literally step back in order to create a larger or different space that is not dominated by one or the other and can be shared. When we think about the Ritchies helping people on the "suicide cliff," we imagine that they were careful not to get too physically close to the person contemplating plunging off the edge lest they startle or provoke, but instead held back a bit, yet *overcame* the distance by beckoning the distraught stranger to their kitchen table.

We can draw nearer to someone in many different ways, great and small. A phone call from the other side of the world, a supportive nod across the room, a handwritten sympathy card, a chair pulled up to the bedside, an embrace. What is possible and what is fitting will vary by the situation and the persons involved, circumstances that determine who is available to welcome, who can achieve proximity, and by what means.

The Covid-19 pandemic that began early in 2020 gave all of us new insights into the importance of proximity and how it can be achieved, about what might be possible and fitting when our usual modes of being with one another are disrupted. Sometimes physical closeness, despite being intensely desired, is not possible, at least from those with whom it is most wanted. What does welcome look like under such conditions?

As the deadly and highly contagious nature of the coronavirus became evident, visitors were barred from most hospitals and could not even be with family members who were dying. In response, many hospitals got creative, using video technology via phones and computer tablets, so that family members could see and be seen by, hear and be heard by their loved ones. It was not the same as being physically present, but it was a fitting and compassionate response to the situation. Note, too, the difference between a voice call and a video call, the latter allowing visible expression and attention—eye contact, smiles, tears, and blown kisses—and, thus, greater proximity, distance further overcome. Hospitals and their staff members who went the extra step of providing screen time between patients and families seem to have understood this important distinction.

Gratitude for such thoughtful creativity is often, and rightly, given to the persons in actual patient rooms holding the tablets for patients and families to visit one another, but the people responding in welcome were not limited to bedside attendants. Compassionate responders also included people whose jobs don't bring them into patient rooms but who advocated for and put in place the policies required to make these actions possible (see Pattern 29). We hope that hospital administrations and staff will continue, in the absence of pandemic conditions, to routinely facilitate such connections for patients who cannot engage with electronic devices without assistance. These new practices were born of the desperation of the times but can be usefully continued and improved for future use—for example, when a family member lives far away and cannot visit at a time of need, or someone is tasked with making medical decisions for a loved one whose condition they cannot quite comprehend without seeing them.

The benefits of virtual proximity notwithstanding, it is clear that bodily proximity remains crucially important in some situations, such as when the one being welcomed is suffering or dying. There are undeniably times in our lives when we have a strong need and desire for the comfort of another human being's physical presence, even a stranger's. Ben Moor, an anesthesiologist, shared the following pandemic story in the journal *STAT*. He, like many others, found it distressing that, because of the precautions necessary to prevent the spread of disease, so many Covid-19 patients were isolated behind closed doors for much of their hospital stay.

> It is on the medical floors that you see signs of the pandemic: countless shelves of bagged PPE [personal protective equipment] for the next shift, nurses in N95 [mask]s, and closed doors—rows and rows of closed doors.

4. Step into the Room

> Behind every door, a person with Covid-19. Alone. We treat them with the few tools we have in our armamentarium—antiviral drugs, the steroid dexamethasone, oxygen—and we wait. They see their nurse periodically. A food service worker comes in three times a day with a tray of food. Other than that, no human contact.[3]

Once Dr. Moor became vaccinated, he began sitting with Covid-19 patients at the end of his day's work—still wearing a mask, visor, gown, and gloves. They were not always his patients; this was volunteer work.

> At first I tried chatting with them, but when someone is breathing 30 times a minute through an oxygen mask, it's difficult to be a great conversationalist. Now I talk to them, hold a hand, get them water, arrange their pillows. Sometimes I just sit there because I have this nagging, incompletely explored belief that just a human presence, someone bearing witness to their ordeal, has value. Afterward, I call the family because they are victims of this virus too.[4]

Ben Moor found a way to be present for patients struggling with and perhaps dying of Covid and for their families. We believe that his "nagging, incompletely explored belief" about the importance of human presence is about welcome. He was open to and moved by the plight of these isolated patients and responded by providing the physical proximity that assured them that another human being wants to be with them, that their particular existence matters, that even in their affliction they remain solidly within the human community.

Even for those not in hospitals, the pandemic offered eye-opening lessons about welcome and the many ways of achieving proximity. Countless virtual gatherings, via Zoom or other meeting platforms, provided enlightening opportunities to negotiate levels of intimacy and expressions of concern and caring when we could not physically reach out and touch one another. Masking taught us so much more than we had known before about how and whether we communicate with our eyes. All of a sudden, the sinister phrase common to crime writing—"the smile didn't reach his eyes"—became a social problem to be solved, as we practiced conveying goodwill, humor, and fellow feeling with our eyes as well as our voices.

A salient lesson from these unanticipated experiments is that bridging distance—coming closer to another person—is basically about attention, openness, and responsiveness, regardless of bodily proximity. It's more about focus and willingness to be present than about hugs and handholding. Embraces, after all, are not ipso facto welcoming; they can also be a way to stifle the other person or avoid a face-to-face encounter.

This recognition of the primacy of *attention and response* over bodily contact enables us to say with assurance that welcome is fully possible not only in situations in which there can be no bodily proximity but also when being physically closer is not wanted by the one we welcome—or, for that matter, not wanted by the one welcoming. Welcome does not depend upon a person's willingness to be literally touched, and a good thing too, since those who shy away from bodily contact are, nevertheless, still likely to want to know that they too are welcome in this world.

Move closer. Enter the room, pull up a chair, write the note, make eye contact, nod to the stranger, return the phone call, make a video call. Take a step, physical or virtual, toward the other person.

Notes

1 The word "proximity" derives from the Latin *proximus*, an adjective that is the superlative form of the word "*prope*," meaning "near." To be *proximus* to someone is to be *nearest* or *right next* to them.
2 This story can also be found in Margaret E. Mohrmann, "Being Mickey's Doctor," in *Attending Children: A Doctor's Education* (Georgetown University Press, Washington, D.C., 2005), 51–77.
3 Ben Moor, "Too Many Covid-19 Patients Face Death Alone. Vaccinated Volunteers Could Change That," *STAT*, January 27, 2021. https://www.statnews.com/2021/01/27/vaccinated-health-care-workers-immunity-spend-time-visiting-covid-19-patients/
4 Moor, "Too Many Covid-19 Patients."

5

Stay Awhile

Once one has moved toward the other person in welcome, it is not time for a hasty retreat. Welcome is a willingness to "stay in the room," to be present and share space, at least long enough to recognize the other person's uniqueness and our responsibilities to them.

The promise of welcome unfolds over time. The movement toward the other person does not complete the obligation of welcome. If welcome means *I want you here*, it cannot mean simply that I want to move toward you. It must mean that I want to share space—again, not necessarily physical space—with you for at least some period of time. We find the metaphors of stepping into the room and staying in the room helpful here: "stepping into the room" gets you into proximity; "staying" allows welcome to grow into full responsiveness.

The powerful potential of "staying" is evident in a scene we describe here from *Philoctetes*, an ancient Greek tragedy by Sophocles:

> Philoctetes, a war hero and master archer, has been abandoned on a deserted island by his fellow soldiers. They have left him to live or die because they cannot stand to hear his cries of pain or smell his open, permanent, fetid wound. He is left in unremitting agony, their rejection absolute.
>
> Nine years later Philoctetes is joined on the island by a young soldier, Neoptolemus, who has been tasked with tricking him into returning to battle by preying on his hopes of rescue. The Greek army needs Philoctetes' help—and his special bow—to win the war against Troy. When Neoptolemus comes upon the older warrior, he finds that, despite the passage of so many years, Philoctetes' suffering is as severe, his wound as festering and horrid smelling, his cries as unbearable to hear, as when he was first exiled.
>
> The generally morally upright Neoptolemus at first goes along with the devious plan to which he has been assigned. But then in a pivotal scene he witnesses Philoctetes succumbing to an extended fit of horrific pain. When

the older man implores him not to leave—"I entreat you, do not leave me alone"—Neoptolemus promises, for himself and the chorus, "Do not be afraid. We shall stay."[1] As his wrenching spasms of pain subside, Philoctetes falls into an exhausted sleep, and Neoptolemus stays by his side. As a result of this experience, Neoptolemus appears to regain his moral compass—to recall the person he thought he was and wanted to be—and aligns himself with Philoctetes against those who would use and abandon him again.

For several years, beginning in 2005, Bryan Doerries brought this central scene to life before numerous audiences of medical professionals as an educational exercise.[2] In this "reader's theater," actors present Sophocles' ancient, timeless drama to the very people likely to be present for such suffering, insisting that they learn to hear it as it comes. The actor playing the role of Philoctetes howls the cries of a once-strong man now stricken with overwhelming pain, laced with the bitterness of betrayal and isolation. There are no words that describe it, nothing that fits into medicine's traditional ways of classifying episodes of pain, including attempts to quantify it on a scale of 1 to 10. There are only the inarticulate, loud, shattering groans of someone whose suffering is beyond bearing. As one of our physician colleagues told medical students about to witness the presentation, it is the kind of encounter that *makes you want to leave the room*.

But Neoptolemus did not leave. He stayed, as he promised. We should be clear here. We are not presenting Neoptolemus as a model of a welcoming person. He didn't decide to stay by Philoctetes' side because he had come prepared to be open and responsive to the old warrior. On the contrary, he had come to deceive him and was in the process of deceiving him when the reality of Philoctetes' deep suffering unfolded before him. It seems to have been less a desire to welcome and more a basic sense of courtesy, followed by a sort of troubled fascination, that kept Neoptolemus riveted to the scene of anguish in front of him. Once there, he was shocked into awareness, his perception of Philoctetes so forcefully ruptured that he changed course, began to recognize his responsibilities to his now friend and, not incidentally, to recall his own moral commitments to himself.

Neoptolemus' act of *staying in proximity* enabled him to open himself to Philoctetes in friendship, loyalty, and responsibility—in welcome.[3] He needed the "wake-up call" that came from his attentive observation of Philoctetes in pain. In contrast, we can so cultivate our welcoming orientation—our openness to being interrupted, changed—that we do not generally require surprise or epiphany to alert us to our responsibilities to others, especially when the others' needs are great (see also Pattern 22). The practices encouraged throughout this book can help us anticipate and prepare to receive the revelation of who the other person is, what they are experiencing, what they may need from us.

In some situations, it may be hard to put a finger on what exactly is or might be accomplished by staying in proximity, especially if we are looking for something tangible or measurable, or even name-able, like Neoptolemus' decision to befriend and ally himself with Philoctetes. How would we name what was accomplished when Ruth, the social worker, sat in the PICU with Mary and her dying child (Pattern 4)? What exactly did Ruth do?

It is not clear that Ruth's returning day after day to sit awhile in the room contributed to any of the things we might imagine—or hope—could result from sitting by a patient's bedside along with family members, like improvements in the patient's well-being or in family members' emotional strength or outlook. Ruth was mostly silent, and when she did speak, she would simply murmur, "I don't know," voicing her inability to comprehend what life was dealing out to Mary and Mickey.

Margaret admits that she didn't immediately grasp what this story might be about. Yet the story stayed with her, and she found that her memory of what Ruth had done for Mary—whatever it was—helped Margaret herself, as a physician and also as a friend and family member, to stay by many more such bedsides. By following time and again Ruth's model of quiet companionship, she came to understand what Ruth was doing and, in working on this book, saw that it could be articulated most clearly in the language of welcome.

Ruth was fully present. She refrained from distracting Mary with meaningless platitudes or pointless questions. In silence, she worked out her own bafflement and sorrow. Each of these is an unquestionably important aspect of what her staying there meant, but the language of welcome allows us to appreciate there is even more going on in this story.

As she sat there, Ruth *opened* herself to Mickey and Mary and allowed herself to be vulnerable to experiencing, insofar as she could, the reality of the dying, the grief, the helplessness. This does not mean that she welcomed Mickey's dying. Welcome is of *persons*—but it is of persons *as they are*. She welcomed Mickey, dying, and Mary, grieving. Encounters with sorrow, vulnerability, and death need not themselves be "welcomed," but welcoming others may well entail bearing their pain with them.

We've said that you may not be able to determine the fitting response to the other person unless you have allowed yourself to stay in proximity with them. But as Ruth stayed in the room with Mickey and Mary, open and vulnerable, she seems not to have discovered a "next step," something to do differently or additionally to help ease their suffering. Except—*except*—Ruth's response was to come back the next day, and the next, predictably and devotedly, to stay with them over time. The "next step" was simply to return, to the end.

This was a most fitting response. Ruth daily, patiently, and steadfastly held Mickey and Mary's new reality with them. In that act of holding, she helped transform the reality, terrible as it was, into a recognizably human experience that *could* be held, that could be endured, an experience that Mary—and perhaps Ruth, too—could live with for the rest of her life, even sometimes with a smile.

Staying can ask a lot of us. Not so much because of the time or inconvenience involved, although these certainly may pose practical barriers to staying. But because when we stay, we make ourselves vulnerable to being changed in some way by this encounter with the person we wish to welcome, whether they are a stranger or someone we've known for a long time. Staying can and should open us even more.

The knowledge that someone is there for you, will stay with you, can make a significant difference in how you experience a troubling time. In the midst of writing this book, Lois experienced a severe and painful eye condition that took months to resolve. In the early stages, the ultimate trajectory was not clear. Would it be full recovery or a cornea transplant, permanent vision loss, or even loss of her eye? She is grateful for the attentive and competent medical care her corneal specialist provided. But what she will most remember is what her eye doctor said on their fourth visit in as many days: "I'm going to get you through this." And she did.

People are to be welcomed as they are, but the welcomer also comes into the act and space of welcome as *they* are, including how they "stay in the room."

> Roz Chast, a cartoonist for the *New Yorker*, has written a remarkable graphic memoir that chronicles her experiences with her aging, then dying, parents. The book ends with the death of her mother, with whom she had a sometimes rocky relationship. Though the entire book is made up of Chast's colorful and frenetic cartoon drawings, including dialogue in bubbles and her own ironic observations, the last few pages contain something else altogether. She has included drawings—not cartoon drawings but penciled portraits—of her mother's face over the summer of her dying and then after her death. Chast sat beside her mother's bed after she died and did what for her was a natural way of connecting: she drew her. Chast writes, "I was alone with my mother's body for a while. I drew her. I didn't know what else to do. I had been drawing her all summer, since the conversations had been reduced to almost nothing."[4]

Someone else might sing, pray, or read poetry in those moments during and following a loved one's death. In a presentation following the publication of the memoir, Chast said she had heard criticism from people about her response. One woman had insisted to her that had it been she, she would have crawled into bed and held her mother's body. But this was clearly not appropriate for Chast and her mother. Such an act would have been so far removed from anything that resembled their relationship in life that it would have been false and forced. Instead, she "stayed in the room" in a way that was authentic to herself and honored her relationship with her mother.

We opened this pattern by stating that the promise of welcome unfolds over time. It is true that sometimes our welcoming encounters are brief, and should be. Lingering in the checkout line to deepen a connection with an unfamiliar cashier not only would seem strained and unnatural but would likely be downright bothersome to the busy cashier and customers standing in line. In many other instances, however, welcome both permits and requires that we stay with another person long enough to develop or fulfill deeper relationships of responsibility. Every situation is different.

For the stranger you meet at a neighbor's backyard barbecue, it may mean that, following introductions, you engage in attentive conversation rather than glancing around to check out who else is there. That's an easy one. And, honestly, when people have asked us about our project, this seems to be the sort of example that first comes to their mind: How do we interact with a stranger in a one-off encounter? Engaging in attentive conversation with someone you've just met *does* fit our conception of welcome. Plus, it's the kind of everyday practice that reinforces deeper commitments to welcome. But it is a limited example that seems little different from common courtesy and does not fully demonstrate the radical openness and responsibility of welcome.

The ethics of welcome we present in this book includes but goes far beyond first-time encounters, as is evident in the stories we have presented in this pattern. They are tales of persons willing to stay and be fully present in a life-altering encounter (Neoptolemus), in sustained daily meetings over a period of weeks (Ruth), and through a lifetime of shared experiences (Roz Chast). We've seen soldiers who go from being strangers to allies, a caregiving professional who steadfastly attends to a patient and family in their worst time of suffering and sorrow, and an artist who expresses her deep love and respect for her deceased mother through her art. Each situation is different, both in how proximity is achieved and in what it accomplishes. Common to each, however, is the human connection established and reaffirmed by staying in the shared space of welcome.

Stay! Listen to the other person's story, their expressions of pain, sorrow, hope, joy. Hold their silence. Stay especially when a person is in need. Express your willingness to stay, if possible. Stay long enough to recognize the next step in welcome.

Notes

1 Sophocles, *Philoctetes*, trans. David Grene, in *The Complete Greek Tragedies*, Vol II, *Sophocles*, ed. David Grene and Richmond Lattimore (University of Chicago Press, Chicago, 1992), 438, lines 805–806, 810.
2 Information about Dorries and the Theater of War projects that grew out of his initial work with *Philoctetes* can be found at theaterofwar.com.
3 This interpretation reinforces the discussion in Pattern 3 of the interchangeable order of "steps" in the process of welcome.
4 Roz Chast, *Can't We Talk About Something More Pleasant?* (Bloomsbury, New York, 2014), 208–22, at 210.

6

Invite the Other Person In

The space welcome creates is shared *space in which each participant is willing to be open not only to receiving but also to offering some degree of self-revelation.*

A medical student wrote of his difficulty getting a history from an 84-year-old woman in a skilled nursing facility. Every question he asked seemed to be met with suspicion. When he introduced himself, holding out his hand to shake hers, she refused it. She asked him how young he was, a question he evaded by saying, "Not too young, I promise." When he began asking questions about her health, she countered, "Why do you keep asking about my poo so much? What's wrong with you?" The physical exam was met with similar resistance.

Even the student's intentional effort to build some rapport by asking what she liked to do in her free time was rebuffed. She barked, "Why? What do you like to do in yours?" The student evaded again, saying "Oh, I don't have much free time." The patient just squinted at him. And then he gave in. He told her that he liked to go to the farmers' market on Saturdays.

That one simple but open reply changed the course of their encounter. She asked him if he ever bought honey there, and when he said "Yes," she replied, "Good!" The student reported that he was going to ask why she said that but, he writes, "I decided to stay quiet instead. It might have been the only correct cue I picked up on in that entire conversation." For, into his now open silence, she began to talk about her honey farming, how honey achieves its taste, how long it matures, and about how she had become a self-taught honey farmer fifteen years earlier when her husband died.[1]

The student was finally allowed to enter his patient's world—not just her world of honey bees and the community college classes she took in her seventies but also, as it turned out, her world of symptoms and a complicated medical history—only when he let her enter his world, even just that little bit. The student's "giving in" to his cranky patient's persistent questioning was the point at which he became truly welcoming. He took a step toward her, a step toward establishing the shared space of welcome within which a relationship of trust can arise.

Thomas Ogletree, in his path-breaking book on Christian understandings of hospitality, wrote, "My readiness to welcome the other into my world must be balanced by my readiness to enter the world of the other."[2] The corollary is equally true: My willingness to enter your world has to be balanced by—and may even depend upon—my willingness to welcome you into my world.

The alternative is to risk becoming nothing but "empathic wallpaper." That's Pat Barker's memorable phrase from her novel *Regeneration*. Billy Prior, a shell-shocked victim of the First World War, accuses W. H. R. Rivers, his psychiatrist, of being just "empathic wallpaper" because he refuses to let any part of himself show. Later on in the novel, Rivers is trying to find out what Prior wants his future treatment plan to be, and Prior says, "I just think you might consider the possibility that this patient might want you to be you."[3]

Of course, the difficulty with letting others into our world is that we have *boundaries*, and rightly so. We can't always easily tell when, if ever, it is appropriate or safe to let them drop, even minimally, or to step around them, even tentatively.

Most of us establish, at a relatively early age and not quite consciously, conditions under which we will share some part of ourselves and our history with someone else, criteria about what someone has to be or to prove in order for us to open up to them, and perhaps different criteria for persons we'll allow to open up to us. Then, we learn—most of us because of continued experience, some of us also because of professional training—to set up even more specific boundaries to cover our new circumstances. The conditions for our willingness to listen, to enter the other person's world, may *expand* as we recognize what our various vocations entail, but the conditions for our opening up to others often *contract*. There are things lawyers just won't tell their clients, teachers their students, or doctors their patients, parts of themselves they won't reveal to persons entrusted to their care. The medical student in the story above, in the process of devising new professional boundaries (a process often only implicitly taught and largely unguided, part of the "hidden curricula" of professional schools), was even reluctant to tell the patient his age.

In general, boundaries are good things. We are almost instinctively wary of people who don't seem to have any; we even label some of them mentally ill. So, to be clear, we are not saying that in order to become welcoming people, we have to become people without boundaries. Rather, as with the many other facets of welcome that require our attentiveness, we must *pay attention to our boundaries*, their existence, their placement, and their purpose.

After all, we set up most of our borderlines, and the rules about if and when they can be crossed, by instinct, before we have much idea of what we're doing. The problem is not that we create them; the problem is that we no longer see them or remember why we put them up. We don't examine them periodically to see whether they still work for us now as well as they did all those years ago when they were put in place. Particularly, we don't remember that *we* put them there—we weren't born with them—and that, therefore, we can choose what we do with them. Even if some of them can't or shouldn't be eliminated, we can still work with or around them as needed.

G. K. Chesterton is credited with this good advice: Don't take down a fence until you know why it was put up. We do not have to tear down our fences in order to be welcoming. But we do have to be aware of them, and we have to question ourselves about them: Why was this fence put up? How and when does it show up in my interactions? What purpose is it meant to serve? Does it actually serve that purpose? Do I still choose that purpose? As welcoming persons, we practice paying attention to the existence of personal boundaries in order to recognize them when we and others hit up against them—What's making me reluctant to engage? What's pulling me away, pushing them away?—and then make a deliberate decision about whether to stay well behind this one, modify it, step around it just this once, or tear it down altogether.

The story told by the medical student of his encounter with the honeybee farmer shows him recognizing, however indistinctly, and then choosing to cross, however desperately, a routine boundary he had set up for himself. The student was able to do a better job of providing care—gathering the patient's history and performing the physical exam—by allowing himself to be known, even if only minimally, and to be vulnerable by being known.

There *are* limits, to be sure. Boundaries, perhaps professional boundaries in particular, serve good purposes. We know of a new mother who had an encounter with a lactation specialist in the hospital that went too far by any standard. Upon learning that the new mother was a professor at the local university, the specialist asked about a currently enrolled graduate student who, she explained bitterly and in detail (while alternately trying to explain how newborns latch on to the breast), had recently had an affair with her husband and broken up her marriage. In another example, a surgeon spent twenty minutes during a presurgical appointment with a lawyer and her six-year-old son explaining how urgently medical malpractice reform was needed in order to limit physician liability. Neither of these examples of "opening up" was appropriate. These professionals were sharing their own preoccupations rather than attempting to forge a bond or create a therapeutic encounter. They needed better, not fewer, boundaries.

It is usually more challenging for us to invite someone into our world than to enter theirs. We certainly have more experience entering the worlds of others. As philosopher Martha Nussbaum has written in *Poetic Justice*, we practice doing that and gain an understanding of actual people when we read literary works and allow ourselves to cheer or cry for imaginary characters. Successful fiction requires us "to see and to respond to many things that may be difficult to confront."[4]

But we don't have as ready a way to practice allowing others into our worlds. And we are often reluctant to do so, hesitant to open up about "things that may be difficult to confront"—sexual practices, for instance, or symptoms of depression or incidents of domestic violence. Hesitation about such fraught issues may extend to more minor personal information—like whether one frequents the farmers' market, or plays tennis, or reads mystery novels—that could give someone at least a glimpse of our hidden selves.

Professionals of various sorts may have higher impediments than most to sharing anything of their worlds. Persons whose work includes potentially high-stakes, intimate encounters with others—clergy and lawyers, for example, as well as nurses and doctors—are often taught, even if implicitly, to place a wall or, perhaps better said, a one-way mirror between them and those who come to them for their professional expertise and assistance. The purpose of this impervious boundary seems to be to keep the professional keenly attentive to the ones seeking help, to make them the priority. But the admonition to stay focused on the other person does not have to be understood as a directive to build stronger walls. It can instead be a guide for navigating with and around one's boundaries: Will sharing this information about myself sharpen or distract from my focus on this person? Will it foster or impede the formation of our shared space? The lactation specialist and surgeon mentioned above violated their obligations of welcome, and consequently their professional responsibilities, with their egregious self-outpourings. In contrast, the medical student's small move of self-revelation, in the story with which this pattern begins, opened the door to more meaningful dialogue with the patient.

If the practitioner does not invite the other person into his or her world, at least partially, while still keeping in mind appropriate personal and professional boundaries, then an asymmetry between the two solidifies. The one who is entrusted with the professional role is too powerful, too distant, and too much "at home" (see Pattern 7), while the one seeking services may feel even more vulnerable, out of place, and perhaps more like an object than a person.

It is important that professionals do not wall themselves off entirely—and the same is true for anyone who wishes to be a welcoming person. Each of us has to strike a balance between having effective boundaries and truly opening ourselves to others, allowing them to know some part of ourselves. Although difficult to learn, this practice of coordinating our limits and our availability, like other welcoming practices, can be cultivated.

To practice welcome is to practice seeking a space to stand with—to live and work and care with—another person. That space cannot be reached without some markers, some borders for the "I" and the "you." But the boundaries cannot be so extensive, so solid and impervious that they cannot be navigated around, penetrated, moved, or re-shaped, as the situation warrants. Attaining that shared space, welcome's homeplace, requires that we find an approach we can live with that is somewhere between having no boundaries at all, on the one hand, and being nothing but empathic wallpaper on the other.

Pay attention to your boundaries; keep them from blocking your ability to be welcoming. As part of your openness to the other person, let them know you, at least a bit.

Notes

1 This story, shared with the permission of Andrew Wang, M.D., a 2013 graduate of the University of Virginia School of Medicine, first appeared in Shepherd, L., Mohrmann, M. "Welcome, Healing, and Ethics," *Wake Forest Law Review* 50 (2015): 259.
2 Thomas Ogletree, *Hospitality to the Stranger: Dimensions of Moral Understanding* (Fortress Press, Minneapolis, 1985), 4.
3 Pat Barker, *Regeneration* (Penguin, London, 1992), 51, 64.
4 Martha C. Nussbaum, *Poetic Justice* (Beacon Press, Boston, 1997), 5–6.

7

Everyone Is at Home

Welcome is a shared space where everyone is at home and has something equally valuable to offer.

This pattern aims to clear up some common misconceptions about an ethics of welcome and further defines welcome by focusing on what welcome is not. In the first pattern, we try to dispel any early impression that being a welcoming person requires one to be an extrovert or to go around seeking people to press one's welcome upon. Our obligation is to welcome the person in front of us. But even the person sitting across from us at the breakfast table or the stranger sitting next to us at the meeting should not have welcome forced upon them. Nor should we consider our welcoming acts as particularly generous when what we are doing is actually obligatory. Welcome is not an exercise of power over another person nor is it a gift, truths that also help distinguish welcome from common conceptions of hospitality.

> A physician was called at 5 a.m. to see an 86-year-old man in the Emergency Department. The doctor, a resident at the time, was bone-tired after almost two weeks of 14-hour night shifts as the internal medicine consultant in the ED. She looked at her elderly patient, "Mr. B.," and saw a stereotype: "I had Mr. B. categorized in a split second. He is going to be from a nursing home. He is going to be demented. He will not be able to give me any history."
>
> As she began speaking with him, some of her pre-judgments were overturned. He lived at home with his wife and was moderately active. His medical history was difficult to put together, but he could answer her questions, if slowly and laboriously.
>
> When she began the physical examination, she warned Mr. B. that her hands were cold. "'Please do whatever you have to, doctor, it won't bother me,' he answered serenely." As she placed one hand on his chest, Mr. B. slowly reached for her other hand. He "started rapidly and vigorously rubbing my

hand between both of his. I stopped my exam to stare at what he was doing. 'To warm you up, doctor. My wife also gets cold when she's tired. This has always helped her.'" He then did the same with her other hand.

"It felt incredibly good, and I continued to watch silently with amazement. He was the sick one, not me. And yet this man, with whom I had been impatient for the past 20 minutes, was concerned about my well-being!" The doctor concluded this brief tale by saying, "It is impossible to convey the feeling of goodness that Mr. B. gave me that morning, but at that moment, it was clearly the patient rather than the doctor who had the healing touch."[1]

The physician/author, Lucie Opatrny, identified her experience as one of healing unexpectedly offered to her, the presumed healer, by her patient, the one assumed to be in need of healing. And so it surely was for her. She had typed him as just another elderly person with multiple problems, like so many she had seen before (see Patterns 10, 13). In contrast, he found something to like (see Pattern 15): He registered her fatigue and cold hands, thought of his wife, who also gets cold when she's tired, and literally reached out to offer warmth and invigoration.

Throughout the book, we speak primarily of and to the one wishing to welcome, but we want to be clear that *in an ideal welcoming encounter, one who welcomes is also being welcomed*. Welcome is a universal obligation owed by everyone to everyone, all the time (certain limits to this responsibility may arise in unusual circumstances explored in Part IV). However, whether welcome is actually offered by each party in an encounter—whether each person accepts and carries out the obligation to be welcoming—is not guaranteed. *Mutual* welcome is rather the *ideal*, for individuals and for communities, the paradigm for human flourishing. Even when the ideal is not fully attainable—as, for many reasons, may often be the case—welcome's *aspiration* toward mutuality can still guide and motivate us as we carry out our moral obligation to be welcoming people.

Welcome Is Not a Gift; It Makes Giving and Receiving Possible

Welcome is our open responsiveness to the other person that allows fitting actions to be undertaken. Some of those ensuing, responsible actions (assistance, affirmation, quiet listening, information-sharing, skilled interventions, and the like) may be construed as gifts, but whether they are labeled as such by either party is not at issue here. Despite theories about what constitutes a "gift,"[2] in ordinary usage the category is a loose one, applied somewhat idiosyncratically. For example, the hand massage in the story above may or may not be considered a "gift" by the doctor, or the patient, or the reader—and we offer no argument either way. Our only insistence is that the patient's welcome, his open responsiveness to the doctor and his effort to overcome the distance between them, is not a gift from him to her but an obligation.

To construe welcome itself as a gift places the welcomer in a dominating position that is antithetical to the nature of welcome as both obligatory and ideally mutual. Rather, what welcome makes possible is a relation—a shared "home"—within which giving and receiving can happen. Within that relational space, we learn a lot about what can and should be given and received. Like the doctor in our story, we become alert to what each of us in this encounter has to offer.

Over the many years during which we supervised first-year medical students as they began learning the skills of interviewing patients, we were frequently confronted by the students' discomfort. Their uneasiness had many sources, including performance anxiety, but almost invariably they insisted upon one primary reason for their disquiet: They had nothing to *give* to the patients because they had not yet learned nearly enough to "play doctor" in any substantive way—that is, they could not give medical information or help. Therefore, they deplored "using" patients solely, as they saw it, for their own educational benefit.

Our responses to their worries covered a lot of territory, including gentle explorations of assumptions about power—power one claims or desires to possess—that are packed into the need to be the identified *giver*. We pointed out the importance of accepting the other person as a contributor and oneself as a recipient. But the practical, and often more effective, part of the reply was to help them grasp just how much they actually were offering the patients. First, we reminded them that each of the patients had volunteered to be interviewed; they did it willingly (some of them more than once during a hospitalization) and in full awareness that the students had little or no medical knowledge. Then we asked the students to think about the fact that serious illness tends to make its sufferers, who are at least temporarily dependent on others for care, feel they have nothing to give anyone. In the face of that, the presence of the students turns the patients into *teachers*, a position of singular authority ("no one knows my illness better than I do") and open generosity ("I will tell you what you need to learn"). Some patients, after such an interview, proudly identify themselves as a "teaching case," the tedious, introspective course of their illness having been converted into a valued opportunity to be of use.

By their focused listening and obvious thirst to learn, the students give the patients their time, attention, and—not to be taken lightly—gratitude. We encouraged students to end each interview by asking the patients what advice they had for them as novices just starting out on the path to becoming a doctor. We never knew a patient to be at a loss for a response to that request and saw the energy and thoughtfulness with which they crafted their reply, another offering from patient to student.

All of this occurs in the context of the students and patients alike practicing some level of intentional open responsiveness toward each other, welcoming each other. Within the relation thus formed, giving and receiving, teaching and learning, respect and affirmation flow freely back and forth—and students and patients alike can see that each has something equally valuable to offer.

Welcome is not itself the gift. Welcome creates the "home" in which the circle of giving and receiving can happen, a circle without beginning or end, in which labels of "giver" and "receiver" blur and blend.

Welcome Is Not an Exercise of Power over the Other Person

An insightful clergyman, known for being warmly pastoral, commented to this effect after reading an early draft of this book: "I may be overthinking this, but with recent events highlighting the issue of White privilege, pervasive racism, and of course the blot of clergy sexual misconduct, I guess I am hypersensitive about welcome becoming patronizing or paternalistic, or at least being perceived as such." He is right. Vigilance on this score is essential.

To begin, welcome cannot be forced on another person. It is not based on an intention to impose oneself on the other person in any way, for any reason. If the doctor in the story above had yanked her hand back when the patient reached out for it, he—if he were truly welcoming—would not insist on grabbing it again. Instead, he would apologize, perhaps with the same words he used about his wife's cold hands as an explanation of his action, and then continue to be open and responsive, alert to other ways in which he can more appropriately express his attentiveness to her.

Welcome is a deliberate opening—a willingness to know and be moved by the other person, a desire to respond fittingly and well to the reality of the other person—not an act of intrusion. It is an aperture, not a probe. If the actions I take to express my welcome are rebuffed (even despite my trying to help the other person welcome me in return, as discussed in Pattern 24), then I stop acting that way.

This doesn't mean I then walk away, or take offense, or do nothing for or with the other person. I am still obligated to be a welcoming person, and I may have other obligations, perhaps professional duties, toward this person that still need to be carried out. Rather, it means either that I have been mistaken in what I thought would be fitting actions or that this encounter cannot approach mutuality, and the shared "home" within which we could come to know each other more fully cannot be formed, at least not yet. (See Pattern 27 for a discussion of maintaining a welcoming orientation even while forgoing particular welcoming actions.)

The realities of racism and sexism, White supremacy and patriarchy, and other routine abuses of power require us to give concentrated attention to how persons we wish to welcome respond to our overtures. Welcome is crucially about paying attention, and one of the aspects of any encounter that most demand our attention is *how we present ourselves and how we are being perceived* (see Pattern 18). My good desire to welcome must include a willingness to examine my own implicit prejudgments and tendencies to stereotype (Pattern 10) that can result in some of my welcoming acts being or appearing condescending or even predatory. Similarly, an ethics of welcome does not allow us to ignore the effects that persisting social injustices and enduring marks of oppression have on the possibility of our welcoming each other across long-standing divides. My desire to be open and responsive to some other person does not of itself erase whatever reasons the other person may have for not trusting me or for preferring not to welcome me in return.

The powerful effects of welcoming and being welcomed in return, of engaging in open and attentive dialogue, are considerable. However, the "power" inherent in welcome is not "power over"—not dominance, presumed supremacy, exploitation—but, rather, "power to," an unleashed capacity for cooperative efforts toward shared goals that can change both lives for the better.

Yielding one's capacity for domination in order to be welcoming does not mean permitting the other person to dominate instead. The exertion of "power over" by *either* party is a serious impediment to welcome because it directs the encounter away from the ideal of mutuality. In contrast, a welcoming person desires to move closer to a situation in which the abilities and attributes of each party are valued and work together to realize the joint purpose of the encounter, whether that purpose is a lesson learned, an illness treated, a project completed, or, most important, the formation of the relationship itself within which all else becomes possible.

Welcome Is Not "Hospitality": Everyone, or No One, Is at Home

Our efforts, in this pattern and elsewhere, to dispel any notion that the welcomer is in a position of superiority or authority over the one welcomed means that we must disentangle the concept of welcome not only from giver-receiver formulations but also from host-guest models. Being the giver and being the host are both positions of authority of a sort: the power to give or withhold at will, to be at home and not a stranger, to appear strong and not vulnerable, to offer something of value and not be seen as in need.

Many of us carry a rather concrete image of what hospitality entails: I am at the door of my house, in the role of host, welcoming you, stranger or friend, as my guest, inviting you to come in. This image is often extended metaphorically to other situations such as classrooms, religious institutions, shops, hotels, and hospitals. Consequently, our customary model of hospitality assumes a host and a guest, a giver and a receiver, a person at home and a visitor welcomed in.

In the face of such an imbalance of perceived status, those who write about hospitality seek ways to soften the inequality between host and guest. Ethicist Thomas Ogletree, for one, asks us to remember how much a guest has to offer. The host in a home setting offers food and drink and a comfortable place to be with others. But the guest, in turn, extends appreciation of what the host has presented. More, the guest offers her stories, her "novelty." Ogletree describes the relationship between the host and stranger as one of shifting asymmetries, in which the host, in their own familiar, safe environment, is both more powerful than the stranger and yet also more vulnerable once the stranger begins to speak: "[W]hen the stranger begins to tell her stories, a new kind of asymmetry appears. With regard to the world of meaning which she is uncovering, she enjoys a level of authority that wholly surpasses my own."[3]

This evocation of what the guest brings to the encounter seems clearly to echo the story with which we began this pattern. The doctor's authority as hosting healer is surpassed by her patient-guest's unexpected expertise not only in regard to his own story but also in his act of healing care. She can only watch in wonder as he warms her hands and soothes her weary impatience.

Both the physician's story and Ogletree's expansive conception of hospitality uncover the mutuality already inherent in the linguistic root of "hospitality." The Latin word *hospes*—the source of "hospitality" and, of course, also of "hospital" and "hospice"—means *both* "host" and "guest." That is, someone who practices hospitality is a *hospes* and, as such, is in both roles, host and guest, simultaneously or alternately. The person standing at the door is a *hospes*, and so is the person standing on the porch, waiting to come in; each is engaging in hospitality. The person I think is my guest is also practicing hospitality toward me. Linguistically, "host" and "guest" are fluid, interchangeable terms.

This rich and playful linguistic ambiguity about who, in any given moment, is the host and who is the guest is a sense of hospitality that we have largely lost. Perhaps nowhere is this loss clearer than in healthcare, where we are usually quite sure of the fixed distinction between host and guest. The hospital (by its very name) is the hospitable one, host to the patients who are its guests. At our university hospital, we have an office of "guest services" responsible for seeing that "guests"—patients and their accompanying family members and friends—have a satisfactory experience during their visit. Persons employed by hospitals, perhaps particularly healthcare professionals and administrators, regard it as their space where they are at home; they are the hosts. Patients are the strangers, come to visit for a while, to receive what the hospital has to offer. And they are expected to behave as guests: not be too demanding, appreciate the food they're served, stay no longer than three days, and say "thank you." It is not surprising that the doctor in the opening story was dumbfounded by her patient's warmth and care because, in the hospital, it is clear who the hosts are and who the guests are and that they're not the same people.

In contrast, then, to the common understanding of hospitality—but entirely in line with hospitality's true meaning—it is the task of welcome to reach beyond the host-guest construct to create instead a space that belongs to no one party individually, but to all conjointly. *An ethics of welcome insists that the world is not divided into hosts and strangers. Everyone, or no one, is at home.*

The shared space that welcome creates—whether in a classroom or a community, a temple or a clinic examining room—is like the overlap of two sets in a Venn diagram. It is where some portion of my world intersects with some portion of yours (see Pattern 6), forming an area, a "home"—temporary though it may be—that belongs to both of us. Not my home with you visiting, nor your home with me intruding. *Our* home for at least the time of this encounter.

Truly open and welcoming experiences with other people decenter us. We are dislodged from our feeling of being the one who is at home—from seeing ourselves as host or giver or authority—into a shared endeavor in which the lines of expertise and influence are no longer clearly drawn. We open ourselves to change, even rupture, of long-held assumptions, to discovering things not only about others but about ourselves that may delight or disturb us.

Welcome makes possible balanced giving and receiving. As you welcome others, do not think of or present yourself as the one who gives or serves as host or sets the terms of the engagement.

Notes

1. Lucie Opatrny, "The Healing Touch," *Annals of Internal Medicine* 137, no. 12 (2002): 1003.
2. The classic example is the work of Marcel Mauss in *The Gift: Forms and Functions of Exchange in Archaic Societies*, trans. Ian Cunnison (Norton, New York, 1967).
3. Ogletree, *Hospitality to the Stranger*, 3–4.

8

Welcoming Ourselves

Welcome is owed to all, including ourselves.

Among the many alterations to our lives caused by the Covid pandemic, our increased use of electronic ways of being together, like Zoom, expanded our understanding of welcome in surprising ways. One participant in a regular group meeting, which switched to gathering virtually during the pandemic, put it this way: "One of the unexpected consequences of using Zoom . . . is that I see not only the community but myself as part of that community." When we meet electronically and look upon the others gathered there, persons we want to welcome and want to be welcomed by, we see *ourselves* in their midst. When we speak to others on the screen, we have to look directly at ourselves in order to make it appear, via the camera, that we are looking directly at them. That's disconcerting, but it's also instructive.

The participant also said, parenthetically, "Is that really what I look like?" Of course, the answer is "yes," but the question is one we're all likely to ask ourselves, usually from a critical, even cringing perspective: Is that *really* what I look like?

> For most of her adult life, Margaret has had the frequent, recurring experience of being called "sir" by people she encounters briefly, by cashiers and clerks, for example, people who are expected to be polite to the public, to say "sir" and "ma'am" or "miss," but who often only glance in someone's direction before deciding which term applies. When this happens, Margaret's habit—not really consciously chosen, but definitely practiced, so a habit—had been to say nothing, just stand there. Almost invariably, the person who called her "sir" would realize the error, get embarrassed, apologize (sometimes over and over), and make some excuse like "It's been a long day." The problem, as she saw it, was not so much being called "sir" in the first place; it was

having to take care of the other person's embarrassment, to suffer through yet another awkward encounter. So, her habitual reaction, she is now sorry to say, had been one of irritation and making that irritation quietly obvious by engaging as little as possible with the person, including pretty much ignoring their apologies. Basically, as she puts it, she pouted and just wanted the encounter to be over.

Writing and thinking about welcome forced Margaret to rethink her reaction. She had long assumed that she was called "sir" because she's tall and wears her hair short. But she has had to recognize that she also carries herself in a not quite classically conventional feminine way. She's sort of androgynous, and she likes being that way—it's who she is, who she is comfortable being.

What she discovered in reflecting on these encounters was that if she wants to be welcoming of others—and has no intention of presenting herself other than as she knows herself to be—then she needs to respond differently to persons who mistake her for a man because they pick up on certain cues that are actually there. Yes, she realized, I really do look like that.

One day, when encountering yet another "sir" from a cashier, followed by his embarrassed apology, she surprised herself by not *reacting* but instead *responding* (see Pattern 2). She made eye contact, smiled, and said, "It's all right." The cashier smiled back, looking relieved. It felt good.

Margaret felt that she was welcoming herself as well as the cashier. And she realized that the lesson learned that day had wider implications: *We cannot welcome others well unless we also welcome ourselves.*

Welcome is a radical, intentional openness to another person, just as they are in that moment. And welcome is a radical, intentional openness to myself just as I am, right now.

This may not be an easy stance for many of us. We are often quite critical of ourselves and may avoid the openness to self that welcome calls for in order not to end up in such a negative place. But an ethics of welcome does not ask that we enjoy or find good every aspect of the person we're welcoming. That's not the work of welcome. We welcome the *person*, the whole person, even if not every detail of what that person says or does. An ethics of welcome insists that we see others as they are and respect them, neither because of nor despite any particular traits they bear, but simply as whole persons who have certain unique characteristics. Just so, an ethics of welcome does not ask that we enjoy or find good every aspect of ourselves. It doesn't speak to whether we do or do not need improving. Rather, it asks that we be *open* to and, thus, aware of who we are—even the uncomfortable things about us, things we might wish were otherwise—and respect ourselves as whole persons, bearing our own particular characteristics.

Welcoming ourselves means acknowledging and owning our shortcomings and blind spots, and the scars we've acquired in living our particular lives. We are who we are. Those of us who grew up with an alcoholic or abusive parent or a pedophilic uncle or who suffered some other sort of life-altering trauma are not likely to escape the long-term effects of those experiences, the damages that we have to work through or around. But we can be aware of and attentive to those aspects of ourselves as we reach out in welcome to others. White persons who grew up in the Jim Crow South are not going to magically rid themselves of the insidious stereotypes of Black persons that permeated their impressionable early years. But they can nevertheless be mindful of the way they have been formed and do the work, every time, of stepping past that formation in order not to be controlled by embedded racist assumptions, in order to be welcoming.

Welcoming ourselves enables us to be aware of our *true* limitations, not only situational constraints of time and energy but enduring gaps in our emotional resources. In Part IV, we consider, in some detail, the risks and costs entailed in being welcoming. One important point made there is that it is possible that a particular individual may be someone I *cannot* personally welcome, not because they are in some way unworthy of being welcomed but because of specific facts about my own life experience (see Pattern 26). It is also the case that the honest self-awareness necessary for that kind of recognition enables me to see when, in truth, I *can* welcome someone whom others may shun.

We don't always know ahead of time what it's going to cost us to open ourselves to a particular person in welcome, and we certainly can't know what it may cost someone else to be welcoming. This is a primary reason why, throughout this book, there is nothing said about welcome and its obligations that is intended or should be used to judge ourselves or anyone for being insufficiently welcoming. The book is about why and how welcome matters and about how we may be able to get better at doing it. It is not about criticizing ourselves or anyone else for falling short of the ideal.

We cannot welcome others well unless we also welcome ourselves. By being open and responsive to who we are—in this moment and in our ongoing lives—not only do we learn how to negotiate accompanying risks but we also become able to recognize and accept the strengths and skills we bring to an encounter. In the previous pattern, and in numerous other instances in the book, we stress the point that all of us often have more to offer, more to bring to challenging encounters than we realize. It is in welcoming ourselves that we discover that, in so many ways, we already have all that we need to be consistently welcoming persons, building communities of welcome and mutual care.

Welcome yourself just as you welcome others.

Part II

Paying Attention

This part of the book encourages perspectives that enable us to see another human being as a whole and unique person, with particular wants, needs, capabilities, and experiences that contribute to making them who they are. Collectively, these practices offer ways of exploring the fundamental question, "Who are you?" (and correlatively, "Who am I?").

9

See a Human Being

First and always, you and I and they are human beings.

In the early 1980s, a delegation of state legislators visited the new pediatric intensive care unit (PICU) at the state medical school's hospital to investigate how state funds were being spent. It was early in the development of specialized intensive care for children. This unit, the first in the state, was an open four-bed ward. The hospital is 100 miles away from the state capital; the legislators chose to travel together in a van. During the trip they shared conversation, snacks, and alcoholic beverages.

At the hospital, the institution's public relations officer gave them a brief orientation then led them into the PICU, where the unit's medical director (Margaret) and nursing staff were prepared to explain the needs of the patients there. The delegates, all middle-aged White men, several of whom smelled strongly of alcohol and were a bit unsteady on their feet, listened impatiently. They handled their apparent discomfort—perhaps they were overwhelmed by the proximity to seriously ill children and the technical means of support crowding the room—by making cracks about "bionic" kids.

Then one of the legislators turned toward the bed of a 6-month-old African American girl with Down Syndrome who was heavily sedated and on ventilatory support after an operation to correct a congenital heart defect. He stared at the infant and said, "Why are we keeping *that* alive?"

Recognizing humanness is essential for an ethics that calls for radical welcome to be offered by every capable human being to every other person, capable or not. We use the terms "human being" and "person" interchangeably. This is intentional; the moral obligations of relation do not allow us to selectively demote certain human beings to nonpersons. Arguments within biomedical and legal ethics that distinguish between human beings and persons are generally tendentious, constructed for the purpose of achieving a desired result (such as rationing resources, justifying the refusal of medical care, or increasing the supply of transplantable organs), and unjustifiable.[1]

Much essential work has been done and continues to be done by philosophers, sociologists, activists, advocates, historians, novelists, filmmakers, legal scholars, and more about the moral requirement to recognize the humanness of others. They explore the biases, unconscious or otherwise, that hinder efforts to do so, and the devastating harms to individuals, communities, and societies that result when this commitment is ignored. We have much to learn. For, unfortunately, we all carry impulses and biases—motivated by self-protection or self-advancement ("us" versus "them" reactions) or by habit, influence, or education—that cause us at times to fail to treat one another with the respect and care that a human being deserves.

Even when the characteristic—race, ethnicity, disability, gender identity, sexual orientation, immigrant status, religious faith, carceral status, and the like—that causes us to see or treat a person as less than fully and equally human is one that we ourselves or our close family members possess, we are not immune to biases against other bearers of that attribute.

The patient in the PICU was a comatose infant. Many health professionals and others who work with very young children, especially premature infants, have grasped the need to deliberately note and remember their humanity, given that these infants may not yet be capable of projecting a clearly human personality that can evoke our spontaneous recognition of their place in the species. Neonatologists sometimes use animal analogies—"skinned squirrels," for one example—to describe how their youngest patients look to them, evidence that recognition of their humanness may not come automatically. The standard and ubiquitous use of the scientific term "neonate" (instead of an ordinary human term, such as baby, infant, child) among health professionals caring for and medical researchers studying preterm or sick newborn children suggests a similar distancing. Even an older infant, if she cannot play the role of a cuddly, laughing baby making eye contact with an adult, may not trigger recognition of her human standing.

The infant in this story also had a noticeable developmental disability. Many of us speak and act as though we believe that persons with well-below-average intelligence are less than fully human. We may prefer to deny such a belief, but our inattention as a society to the actual needs of such persons, our common presumptions about the burdens of caring for such a child, and our overt dread of falling into such a state ourselves reveal our distancing, discomfort, and even disdain.

Conscious, intentional recognition of humanness is a crucial task not only in the neonatal and pediatric intensive care units and in programs for the developmentally disabled but also in encounters with persons of any age who are minimally conscious, in a "vegetative" state (a designation that not only de-humanizes, but even de-animalizes the person), have some form of dementia, or in other ways exhibit a marked diminishment of their cognitive capacities. Such persons may not be able to behave or express themselves in ways common to most human beings, or thereby arouse in us the sort of fellow feeling upon which awareness of our moral obligations toward them tends to depend. Recurring claims that it would be ethically acceptable, even good, to use some such persons as sources of transplantable organs or as unconsenting research substrate reveal how easy it is to "forget" that they are and continue to be fully human. They issue the same moral call on us for respect and fitting care as do all other human beings—all other persons, all other members of the human community—no matter the extent or irreversibility of their differences from those of us who, at least for the time being, appear to possess rational judgment and agency.

The patient was African American. White European Americans have a long, terrible history of regarding non-White persons, especially persons of African descent whose ancestors were enslaved in the United States, as "sub-human" and thereby excluded from the human moral community and its obligations of regard. In her book *Medical Apartheid*, Harriett Washington lays bare the medical establishment's repeated exploitation, from colonial times onward, of Black patients for human experimentation without their knowledge or consent. What made this possible, perhaps inevitable, was the dehumanization of Black people. Among many other examples evidencing this fact, Washington recounts how, in a speech given in the 1960s at Tulane Medical School, a neurosurgeon reminisced about the days when it was cheaper for researchers to use Black patients than cats because Black people (he used a racial slur) "were everywhere and cheap experimental animals."[2]

Overt labeling of Black persons by White persons or others attempting to assert their superiority, in ways that define them as less than human, may not be as common as it once was. We hope, perhaps naively, that a White lawmaker today would be unlikely, even when intoxicated, to speak as the man did in the story with which this pattern begins. Yet racism remains pervasive, its roots deep. Ibram X. Kendi writes in *How to Be An Antiracist* about his realization that, although he is African American, as a child he had internalized racist views of Black people and, as a young man, "wanted to be Black but didn't want to look Black"[3] and preferred dating lighter-skinned Black women. Kendi insists that to be a person who rejects racism—and, we add, who rejects the many other forms of prejudice that prevent us from recognizing the full humanness of others—"requires persistent self-awareness, constant self-criticism, and regular self-examination."[4]

Regardless of whether the labeling is explicit, racial bias—conscious or not—continues to haunt many encounters. We know from multiple investigations[5] that even today, Black patients are less likely to receive adequate treatment for pain or to be considered agents capable of participating fully in decisions about their care.

The patient was a girl. The sorry history of regarding human females as less-than-complete human beings—or "failed males," as long-discredited but tenacious beliefs about fetal development would have it—with inherently inadequate capacities for rationality, ethical behavior, and effective autonomy is well documented and need not be belabored here. Though we must note that, at the time we are writing, hard-won gains in legal equality for girls and women in the United States are being eroded by heightened surveillance and restriction of their medical and other choices when they are or may be or even may become pregnant. Scholars in the last decades of the twentieth century presciently warned about increasing rates of forced Caesarean sections and other coercive interventions, the justifications for which treat pregnant girls and women not as full persons but instead as "incubators" or "fetal containers."[6] The patient in the PICU is only a child, but the dangers of a perspective that grants value to an entire sex primarily or solely on the basis of reproductive ability redound to its younger members as well.

It is irrelevant to our point whether gender-based or race-based disregard and discrimination came first in human history or which is the more fundamental oppression. Gender bias and racial bias are both persistent, often mutually reinforcing temptations (or, for some, reasons) to misjudge the human standing of another person and thus to ignore obligations of respect, care, and welcome. So, too, with other characteristics for which people face unjust discrimination.

Human community is universally inclusive and, therefore, far more extensive than the various historical, geographic, and tradition-based communities that are the focus of communitarian thought.[7] The obligations entailed by our human community call to us prior to the formation of these more narrowly conceived communities—and also prior to particular relationships of care. The ethics of care provides crucial elucidation of moral responsibilities within the borders of particular personal or societal relationships.[8] However, when we speak of welcome, we are focused on *the relation that comes before the relationship*. Welcome is owed to strangers, to those we have just met, and to those we have known for a long time. It is the perception of our common humanness that calls us to look—and listen—again, seeking to know and to respond well to this other person.

A welcoming interaction may result in a continuing or deepening relationship that will benefit from the insights of an ethics of care. It may draw the other person into our particular community or us into theirs, within which we may be helpfully informed by a communitarian ethic. Or we may go our separate ways, stopping short of establishing or continuing an enduring relationship but nevertheless having honored our own and each other's humanity by our mutual recognition and moral responsiveness.

What was her name? Throughout this pattern, we have referred to "the patient" or "the infant" in the PICU, introduced in the opening story. This language, especially in repetition, does not seem very welcoming. When working on this pattern, we wondered if readers would notice this distancing language and if they would be uncomfortable with it. *We* became uncomfortable with it as our exploration kept returning to her, knowing that attention to names is an important welcoming practice (see Pattern 17). Even though we actually don't know her name and could not share it if we did because of patient privacy, it seems we might have honored her in this expanded retelling of her story by giving her a name to emphasize her distinct humanness. However, we chose not to do so for a reason: In this pattern—in this pattern alone—her unique name is not the point. We are asking for the bare ethical minimum here, so let us call her *Human*.

In the following pattern and others, we go much further than this minimum because the simple perception of humanity, although crucial, is not enough. In fact, it can leave us vulnerable to two related errors: first, having seen our common identity as human, we may ignore salient differences between us, and second, the differences we do note may lead us to identify the other person as a distinct "type" of human being. Each error is a way of blinding ourselves to who this particular human being actually is. Welcome requires that we let the other person tell and show us the whole and unique person they are, rather than allowing us to rely simply on our shared humanity to understand what they feel or want or need, or to assign them to a category or type of person we think we already know. There's a tension here because we all *are* of a type: the human type. As we assert in the next pattern, welcome requires that we *recognize* humanness but *acknowledge* uniqueness. There is much further work to be done.

And so now, as we move forward, we can name the human child in the PICU. We name her *April* for the openness of welcome and what is to come.

Recognize that the person we welcome is fully human. Look beyond the absence of familiar cues; examine and step around the presence of contrary biases.

Notes

1 By emphasizing the category of human being/person, we in no way intend to exclude nonhuman animals from moral consideration. We are addressing in this book interhuman relations only, but without prejudice against the claim that human beings also carry significant moral obligations toward the nonhuman animals with whom we share this world.
2 Harriet A. Washington, *Medical Apartheid* (Anchor, New York, 2008), 10.
3 Ibram X. Kendi, *How to Be An Antiracist* (Random House, 2019), 109.
4 Kendi, *How to Be An Antiracist*, 23.
5 See, for example, Kelly M. Hoffman et al., "Racial Bias in Pain Assessment and Treatment Recommendations, and False Beliefs about Biological Differences between Blacks and Whites," *PNAS* 113, no. 16 (2016): 4296–301; and Institute of Medicine, *Unequal Treatment: Confronting Racial and Ethnic Disparities in Health Care* (National Academies Press, 2003).
6 George J. Annas, "Pregnant Women As Fetal Containers," *Hastings Center Report* 16, no. 6 (1986): 13–14, https://doi.org/10.2307/3562083.
7 See, for example, works by Alasdair MacIntyre and Michael Sandel. For a concise introduction to communitarianism, see the 2024 essay by Daniel Bell in *The Stanford Encyclopedia of Philosophy*, https://plato.stanford.edu/entries/communitarianism/.
8 See, for example, works by Virginia Held, such as *The Ethics of Care: Personal, Political, and Global* (Oxford University Press, New York, 2007), and Nel Noddings, such as *Caring: A Relational Approach to Ethics and Moral Education* (University of California Press, Oakland, 2013).

10

See *This* Human Being

Sharing a common humanity does not mean that we are alike in all the ways that matter. Each person we welcome is unique, with their own particular way of being in the world.

As discussed in Pattern 9, *recognizing* the other person as fully human is imperative; no welcome is possible without it. However, it is also important to be keenly aware of certain dangers inherent in the act of recognition. For one, there's the risk of being so convinced of our human alikeness that we slip past our differences into the error of seeing the other person as just "another me," rather than as the irreducibly unique person they are. "Human like me" easily and unwittingly elides into "human in the same way that I am human, experiencing life as I do, making choices I would make." We may be most likely to make this error when we encounter persons who really do seem to be "like us" physically and culturally. However, it also happens when the other person is obviously not "like us," but we deny the importance of the differences.

A second, related peril inherent in the act of recognition is that it may encourage us not just to see a fellow human being but to place that person within a particular subset or *type* of humanness, a form of being human that we "recognize" when we see it.

Larry Palmer, a retired law professor who is Black, has written about what it feels like not to be seen for who he is. Palmer attends a progressive Protestant church. Despite his many years of participation, he is repeatedly mistaken by White congregants for one of the two other Black men who also attend church there regularly. This happens although one of the men is a decade, the other *three* decades younger than Palmer, and it sometimes happens even when he is wearing his church nametag on his jacket lapel. The lapse is all the more striking because, he writes, he does know the names of those who misidentify him, whether they are wearing their name tags or not.

The White churchgoers' inability to distinguish among the Black men is such a routine occurrence that, shortly after President Trump's inauguration in 2017, one of the younger men jokingly asked Palmer, "How are things going for you and Michelle since leaving the White House?"

In the essay in which he recounts this experience, Palmer writes: "This private humor between two blacks in a predominantly white setting hides hurt and anger, indeed seething outrage—a form of distancing from fellow worshippers that is the antithesis of community building."[1]

Growing up, Larry Palmer had heard the adage that "white people think all black people look alike," but writes that he neither believes nor accepts that White people are incapable of distinguishing among Black people who look nothing like each other except for the color of their skin. Instead, he explains the misidentification problem he experiences by reasoning that his White fellow parishioners don't bother to look him or the men he is mistaken for in the face and see their "individual distinctiveness."

Perhaps the White congregants do look, briefly, at his and the other men's faces, but it is likely that they then look away, having seen "enough." Instead of truly seeing and connecting with each man face-to-face, they see enough to put the men in a category in their mind, perhaps the category of "one of the three Black men who go to church here."

Categorizing people we encounter is a rather common human activity. Most of us are likely able to identify an overly needy person, a chronic complainer, a control freak. Healthcare professionals quickly "recognize" certain types: the elderly person with dementia, the drug-seeker, the "worried well." Consider, too, that an assigned type need not be negative, derogatory, or distancing. It can appear to be positive, appealing, well-intentioned. Nurses and doctors, for example, usually respond positively to a patient they understand to be a "sufferer" or, more broadly, when they identify patients as gruff but endearing grandpas, adorable children, and sweet little old ladies. In many ways, such categorizing seems a savvy and efficient thing to do. So, what's the problem?

The problem is that, even when relatively affirmative, categories are inescapably reductive—and they impede welcome. The "LOL in NAD" ("little old lady in no acute distress," a dismissive designation long used in medical charting that we hope is now part of medicine's past) is a common example of vapid stereotyping—in this case of an older woman who does not appear to be at immediate risk of dying—that is far from innocuous. Health professionals using that label may be fond of so-called "little old ladies," but studies have shown that older women are the ones least likely, among hospitalized patients, to have their interests or their wishes taken seriously.

Recognizable types that seem to beckon us closer and stimulate us to care harbor the same risk as those that push us away. Whatever the human pattern identified and whether the identification moves us toward or away from the other person, *the problem arises when we stop there, satisfied that we have classified and now, therefore, know this person*—or, at least, satisfied that we have seen and heard everything we need to know: You are (only) a drug-seeker, or a cute kid, or an obese diabetic, or one of the Black men in the congregation. But recognition is not knowledge, and recognition alone is not enough for welcome.

In Pattern 2, we introduced Count Rostov, the protagonist of Amor Towles' novel, *A Gentleman in Moscow*. His thoughts helped make our point there about the difference between reactions and responses. Here we recall Rostov's musings to buttress the distinction, framed now in different but obviously related terms, between recognition and what's needed to begin to know another person.

> What can a first impression tell us about anyone? . . . By their very nature, human beings are so capricious, so complex, so delightfully contradictory, that they deserve not only our consideration but our reconsideration—and our unwavering determination to withhold our opinion until we have engaged with them.

The engaging work of welcome moves beyond *recognizing* common humanity and "types" of persons to *acknowledging* this particular, one of a kind person. It is this person—not their generic descriptors, real or imagined, positive or negative—whom we want to welcome and to whom we must respond. If recognition can be thought of as a step toward the other person, acknowledgment is a small step back, granting space that allows the other person to speak himself, to say, "I am. This unique way of being that I am exists." Acknowledgment thus makes knowledge of another person possible.[2]

This intentional space is the distance we require if we are to focus clearly on the other person, to see them rightly, as they are, here and now (recall from Pattern 1 that welcome is openness to others *as they are*). Seeing someone rightly is the essential element and, etymologically, the root definition of *respect*.

The philosopher Immanuel Kant said that, while the principle of mutual love always draws us nearer to each other, the principle of mutual respect keeps us at a distance from one another.[3] This does not mean that love (or welcome) and respect oppose one another. Rather, it indicates that respect is an essential companion of love (and of welcome), negotiating closeness and distance in order to bring each of us into focus so that we may be truly known to each other. The moving dance of love and respect, closeness and distance, is a fundamental characteristic of welcome.

Acknowledgment always necessarily precedes knowing. We cannot know a person we have not acknowledged, a person who is still only a recognizable type to us. Without acknowledgment, any "knowing" we think we have gained is likely to be distorted and false, our own invented story about someone we have not truly encountered.

Not knowing something about a person is not a moral failing in itself. Large deficits of information are a given when we meet someone for the first time; some of the gaps may or may not be filled by further interaction and observation, but ignorance is at least potentially remediable. On the other hand, not acknowledging a person as they are in that moment of encounter is significantly more problematic morally. Ethicist Richard Miller has put it this way, citing the philosopher Stanley Cavell: "Our failure of knowledge denotes an absence, a form of ignorance, an epistemic deficit. Our failure of acknowledgement is, in contrast, 'the presence of something, a confusion, an indifference, a callousness, an exhaustion, a coldness.' Seen in this way, knowledge is to ignorance as acknowledgement is to apathy."[4]

Welcome calls us to move from recognition to acknowledgment so that we may know one another more fully in our uniqueness. As always, then, welcome calls us to *pay attention*, and yet more careful attention to the person before us. What might such further attention entail? Count Rostov insists that human beings, in all our delightful complexity, deserve not only consideration but *reconsideration*. Various modes of reconsideration are explored in depth in Part III. But before getting there, in what comes next we continue describing strategies to overcome the impediments that may stand between those who wish to welcome and those they are welcoming.

Acknowledge the persons you welcome as unique individuals so that you may come to know them as they are and as they want to be known.

Notes

1 Larry I. Palmer, "Call Me By My Name," *Blackbird* 17, no. 2 (2018), https://blackbird-archive.vcu.edu/v17n2/nonfiction/palmer-l/call-page.shtml.
2 For this point and what follows, we are indebted to Richard Miller's insightful discussion in the introductory chapter of his *Friends and Other Strangers: Studies in Religion, Ethics, and Culture* (Columbia University Press, New York, 2016).
3 See Miller, *Friends and Other Strangers*, 5. In the Introduction, we make a brief point about welcome being "closely linked with love, especially as love is understood by traditions of thought that emphasize an obligation to love one another as a primary ethical precept." Thus, we draw upon arguments that have been made about the nature and obligations of love to deepen the discussion of welcome.
4 Miller, *Friends and Other Strangers*, 3, quoting Stanley Cavell, "Knowing and Acknowledging," in *Must We Mean What We Say? A Book of Essays* (Cambridge University Press, New York, 2002), 264.

11

Who Is This Person *Right Now*?

Welcome requires paying attention to who people are now, in the moment of our encounter, whether they are a stranger or someone we've known well over a long time.

Because the persons we encounter are whole and complex, much more than the type-defining characteristics we first notice, welcome asks us to reconsider who they are by being curious and imaginative, asking them to tell us who they are, being aware of the fables we concoct about them, and being willing to imagine alternative stories that help us welcome them (strategies discussed in Pattern 15). By doing these things, we can begin knowing *this* person and, therefore, begin to learn the form our welcome is to take and the contours of our responsibility to them.

Throughout, we have reiterated that we are to welcome the other person as he is, as she is, as they are. But more particularly, welcoming someone means opening ourselves to them *as they are right here and now*. Who they are in this moment of encounter with us—not who they are generally or historically or ideally—determines our immediate responsibility to them. This demand is less about discerning some specific thing they may need from us in the moment, although clearly that may be important to learn, than about being broadly aware of their present situation and its call to us to meet them where they are.

In the news article that told of the welcoming work of the Ritchies, the "Australian Angels" who saved many from suicide (see Pattern 1), there is also reported this contrasting tale:

> Kevin Hines wishes someone like Ritchie was there the day he jumped off the Golden Gate Bridge in 2000. For 40 agonizing minutes, the then-19-

year-old paced the bridge, weeping, and hoping someone would ask him what was wrong. One tourist finally approached—but simply asked him to take her picture. Moments later, he jumped.

Hines, who suffers from bipolar disorder, was severely injured but eventually recovered. Today [in 2010] he says if one person had shown they were not blind to his pain, he probably would never have jumped.[1]

The tourist seems to have recognized Kevin Hines as a human being who might be able to operate a camera but to have gone no further than that first impression. She appears to have been blind to his tears, his pacing, his anguish. *Willfully* blind—regardless of whether she made a conscious choice to ignore the signs of his distress—because her will, her intention (part of the basic meaning of welcome) was not prepared to see this young man exactly as he was, right there and then, and to respect and welcome him. It seems she saw a convenient shutter clicker but did not see Kevin Hines, a unique person in distress and in critical need of a response.

What if, as she walked toward him, she had chosen to open herself to him, even just a bit, and had looked at him rightly, with respect? If she had done so, she could not have failed to see him as he was at that moment and thus to register his misery. No longer "blind to his pain" but prepared to welcome him, she could then have chosen to respond to him as he was by saying something like, "What's wrong? Are you okay?" Hines said, in retrospect, that if just one person had done such a thing, had acknowledged him and his turmoil, he probably would not have jumped from the bridge. This is striking testimony to the power of even the most minimal, tentative moves toward welcoming someone.

The tourist's failure does not lie in her ignorance of whatever was tormenting Hines. She may not have been able to sense that he was contemplating jumping from the bridge. As discussed in Pattern 10, ignorance of others is a given on first encounters and not a moral failing. Rather, the problem lies in her failure to *acknowledge* him. She did not pay attention to Kevin Hines, and whether her failure stemmed from awkwardness or preoccupation, or even from indifference or callousness, the result was the same. Had she been open to acknowledging Kevin as he actually was in the moment, she would probably have prevented his plunge from the bridge.

11. Who Is This Person Right Now?

In much of this book, we speak of encounters between strangers, like Kevin Hines and the tourist, or near-strangers, like doctors and their patients. But welcome must also be practiced between persons who already know each other, even within families and close friendships. In fact, the reminder that who someone is *now* matters most may be particularly necessary within already-formed relationships, in which it is so easy to fall back on what we already know, or think we know, and fail to recognize who this person is in this present moment and what their call to us is right now.

Both of these points, about welcome within families and about focusing on who the person is now, were brought home to us one evening during a conference devoted to the concept of welcome developed in this book.[2] Participants were asked to bring to an informal evening session their stories about welcome—times when they felt welcomed or not, times when they thought they had offered welcome or not. The tales were revealing in many ways, not least in the diversity of memories stimulated by the topic of welcome, and we found our understanding of welcome significantly expanded by what we heard that evening. Perhaps most gripping, and most unexpected, were a couple of stories about childhood experiences that the adult narrators now construed as times when they did not feel welcomed within their own families.

> One participant, whom we'll call Michael, said he wanted to talk about how we welcome children, then told his story: About sixty years before, when Michael was nine years old, his mother was seriously injured in an automobile accident. She went through a month of steady recovery, then hemorrhaged into the subdural space around her brain, resulting in paralysis and loss of speech. Michael and his older brother were part of the group that kept vigil at the hospital, along with members of his extended family and the minister from their church, but, he said, "nothing was ever talked about to my brother and me." He expressed his gratitude for the "good things" that happened—including the near-miraculous recovery of his mother, who lived to be 93—but his enduring impression of that frightening time was that it was full of busy experts and of things he didn't comprehend. Michael told us that he has carried "the residuals" with him through most of his adult life. He felt most keenly that he had "no way to put words to it," to articulate either his terror or his gratitude, and no one helped him find the words. He concluded his story by saying "We need to do better for our children."

A bit later in the evening, another participant, "Cory," told this story: Sometime in the 1950s, Cory and his brother underwent tonsillectomies on the same day. After their operations, they were put in adjoining beds in a big ward, but soon Cory's brother began vomiting blood. Medical personnel appeared, moved his brother to another part of the room, and "worked on him through the night." The next day the boys' father came for Cory and, as the two of them were leaving the hospital, Cory asked where his brother was. His father replied, "He's in heaven with the angels." Cory related that he was not part of the funeral, was left alone for the most part, and was not counseled. He was quick to say this was not an indictment of his parents, who he thought did the best they could. But, he concluded, "as a six-year-old child, I didn't feel welcomed into that situation."

Nine-year-old Michael and six-year-old Cory were not welcomed *as they were then*, as young children, reasoning with limited vocabularies and a paucity of concepts. Each of them may well have wondered what he'd done to cause this catastrophe, what would happen to him, where in the world he fit now that everything had changed so radically. But their questions and fears went unnoticed, unarticulated, and unaddressed. The adults responsible for the boys failed to respond to them as they were at that moment—developmentally, rationally, and emotionally immature, and wholly inexperienced in the odd workings of pain and grief.[3]

That the adults in these situations were likely lost in their own emotional turmoil may explain their inattention to the children, and some may think that it's too much to ask of them to step away from their grief and fear enough to focus on the children's needs for explanation and reassurance. However, consider that, many decades after the events had taken place, Michael's and Cory's distress was unmistakable as they spoke of the haunting and persistent pain that resulted from their not being welcomed within their own families at the time when they most needed to be. The adults' failure to welcome them may be understandable, but it was nevertheless a failure with significant, lasting consequences. The adults' feelings, intense as they were, did not absolve them of their responsibilities to and for their children, their obligation to help the children walk with them on the hard path of loss and sorrow, not in aloof silence but in the safe embrace of caring, responsible, age-appropriate welcome.

Who someone is *now* is what matters most as we move to welcome them. The evening session at the conference that called forth Michael's and Cory's narratives of childhood grief and confusion evoked another story that, in contrast, exemplifies welcoming someone as they are, right here and now.

> "Mara" spoke of the recent death of her grandmother when, Mara said, "I got to be the welcoming force in her life." Mara had participated in her "spunky" grandmother's care as she aged, assisting her mother who was the primary caregiver. At the time of the events in Mara's story, her mother was incapacitated by a broken hip, and her grandmother was in a rehab hospital after a bout of pneumonia. When her grandmother developed unremitting pain from a pre-existing, untreatable abdominal problem, she was taken to the hospital where Mara worked as a nurse, and it was Mara who "welcomed her from the ambulance" and then acted as her advocate. Mara worked with the medical team to be sure that her grandmother's pain was relieved and to postpone further testing until the next day so she could rest quietly.
>
> Once she was certain that her grandmother was comfortable and stable, Mara went home for the night. She was called back just a few hours later because her grandmother's condition had changed. Mara said that when she saw her it was clear that she was nearing death. "I knew my grandmother, and I knew she was ready," was the way Mara described her certainty that there should be no medical interventions from that point. Mara asked her if she was in pain; her grandmother shook her head, but was unable to speak. Then Mara lay down in her grandmother's bed and held her, prayed with her ("I knew that would be important to her"), and spoke words of love and release. "We talked about the angels coming to take her. I got to be part of that sacred moment . . . It was my opportunity to help her welcome death."

Mara told this story as one about helping her grandmother welcome death, but we recognize it as the tale of Mara welcoming her grandmother precisely as she was in that moment. Mara saw that who she was *then* mattered most: unquestionably dying and unquestionably still the whole person Mara had known and loved for so long, the person who Mara knew would find profound comfort in being held, in prayer, and in assurances of an angelic escort through death.

The details of what welcome asks us to say or do in response differ according to who the person we welcome is in that moment. Mara's deep knowledge of her grandmother anchored her confidence that her grandmother would find solace and peace in Mara's embrace and prayers, but what Mara did for her grandmother is not a prescription for what every dying person wants or needs. Someone whose affection for their children or grandchildren has never been expressed very physically might find a full-body embrace by one of them at the time of death unsettling and intrusive, just at the time when they most want tranquility. See, for example, the discussion of Roz Chast's choice to sketch her mother as she was dying, an action entirely in keeping with what Chast knew about her mother (Pattern 5); getting in bed to hold her mother would have been a violation of both her mother's integrity and the truth of their relationship. That is, what we've come to know over time about who someone is surely must significantly affect our comprehension of who this person is now, in this moment, and thus shape our perception of how we are to respond to them.

Atul Gawande recounts a story told to him by a palliative care physician, Dr. Block, whose father—an emeritus professor of psychology, researcher, and author—required an operation that carried a significant risk of leaving him with severe neurological damage.[4] Dr. Block would be the one to make medical decisions for him if he were incapacitated, so she had a conversation with her father about his wishes, a talk she went into assuming that he would likely not want to live if he could not continue his treasured academic work. She was astonished when her father said, "if I'm able to eat chocolate ice cream and watch football on TV, then I'm willing to stay alive." She didn't even know he liked football. As she said, "The whole picture—it wasn't the guy I thought I knew." But it was the guy he was right there and then. She had invited him to tell her who he was at that moment, in that situation, and then let that new understanding guide her future decisions.

When encountering someone for the first time, pay attention to the cues that can help you see them as they are in that moment. When interacting with someone you know, draw on your well-established knowledge but also pay close attention to who they are right now.

Notes

1 "Australian 'Angel' Saves Lives at Suicide Spot," *CBS News*, June 14, 2010, https://www.cbsnews.com/news/australian-angel-saves-lives-at-suicide-spot/.
2 Margaret Mohrmann, "'Weave Us Together': The Obligations of Welcome in Clinical Practice and the Moral Life," Medicine and Ministry of the Whole Person Annual Conference, Kanuga Conference Center, Hendersonville, NC, November 2–4, 2018, on compact disc recorded and produced by PhotoVision, 2018.
3 James Agee's autobiographical novel, *A Death in the Family* (McDowell, Obolensky, New York, 1957), presents poignantly and incisively this issue of children's bafflement and adult inattention in the face of death.
4 Atul Gawande, *Being Mortal: Medicine and What Matters in the End* (Henry Holt & Co., New York, 2014), 183–5.

12

Empathy Is Not Enough

There are perils in trying to know another person by imagining how they feel or experience life, even when we mean well. Welcome and empathy call for different strategies for knowing and connecting with another person.

A former colleague of ours, a rehabilitation specialist, asked one of his patients to talk with medical students about how she had adapted to her physical disability. The specialist thought the patient had exhibited exceptional bravery and fortitude in living with her disability and thought his invitation would be appreciated. Instead, the patient rebuked the physician. She was happy to talk to the students about her disability, but she wanted no talk of heroism or exceptional courage. She was an ordinary person like everyone else, facing daily challenges of living.

While this incident happened many years before our friend's telling of this story, it clearly made a deep impression on him. What he told us he learned from this patient was that seeing her as doing exceptionally well in light of her disability was just as patronizing as seeing her as suffering from it, when neither was how she experienced her life.

This pattern explores the dangers of relying too much on our imagination to try to know another person, even if that strategy is prompted by empathy or compassion. Elsewhere (see Patterns 3 and 4), we note that having empathy toward another person does not necessarily result in responsive action. We may *feel* empathy but fail to *act* in any meaningful way. This pattern explores a different way in which empathy may be insufficient. We may think that through our empathetic imagining we understand what another person is experiencing when we really do not. Our internal feelings of empathy may indeed move us to act, but we don't act responsibly because we have misjudged the fitting response as a result of looking inward to our imagination rather than outward to what the other person is showing or telling us, or might be willing to show or tell us if invited.

Empathy is a concept that we both appreciate and interrogate in this book. It is generally understood as the capacity to sense or understand what another person is experiencing, usually through imagining and appreciating how we might feel if we were in that situation, if we were "in their shoes" or "saw the world through their eyes"—common expressions used in descriptions of empathy. Some scholars distinguish among empathy, compassion, and sympathy, and there may be good reasons to do so in some contexts, but we use them interchangeably. The distinctions are not agreed upon and do not bear on the main points we wish to make here about the differences between an ethics of welcome and ethical approaches that rely on any of these generally morally good feelings, each of which involves some measure of reliance on imagination in responding to another's situation. With each, there is both a cognitive element (understanding what a person may be feeling) and an emotional element (sharing in those feelings—"compassion" in its original Latin root means "experiencing or suffering with").

Empathy is considered important for practitioners within most professions that include caring for others in some fashion such as mental health counseling, faith leadership, and teaching. Within the medical and nursing professions, there is strong emphasis on developing one's capacity for empathy in order to establish therapeutic relationships and respond to patients with due care. In fact, the development of empathy is cultivated in children by parents and teachers from early childhood onward. We expect everyone to have empathy.

The impulse is a good one. It means we have a real awareness of and concern for the other person. Although we do not know what it is like to be them, we know what it is like to be human, and as humans, we share much in common.[1] When we experience empathy, we care, and we are trying to understand.

At the same time, relying on empathy to determine right actions can be simplistic, misguided, and even presumptuous. When our empathetic imagining leads us to assume we know how someone feels, rather than actually finding out, we can misjudge what they may need or want and how best to relate to them.

Margaret has written about this problem in an earlier book in which she reflects on her experiences as a pediatrician:

> [I]t is one thing to be able, after careful listening and observation, to say, "I understand what you've let me know about how you feel," and to let that understanding deepen and guide one's relationship with the patient from then on.... However, it is quite another thing, a dangerous and fundamentally immoral move, to proceed from such an understanding, important as it is, to the claim "I know how you feel"—surely the one statement that should be forbidden to all medical practitioners. From that false claim it is but an easy slide to an even more perilous assertion: "Therefore, I know what you want (or need)."[2]

No matter how well-meaning we are and how hard we try to do empathy right, we sometimes need reminding that we are separate persons, separate *unique* persons (see Pattern 10). This means we each necessarily view the world, including the world of the other person, always *through our own eyes*. The lens through which we engage in empathetic imagining is colored by our own life experiences, understandings, and values, including (though we might wish it were otherwise) aspects of ourselves that may not rise to complete awareness because they involve unexamined fear, regret, shame, or loss. Thus, perhaps counterintuitively, empathy can be surprisingly *self-referential*. After all, empathy involves understanding a fellow human being's needs and desires by considering what *my* needs or desires would be if I were in their situation: How would *I* feel if I were lonely or in pain or suffering a loss such as theirs? What if that happened to *me*?

There is an additional drawback to empathy besides the misjudgments we may make in imagining the other's situation. It has to do with the emotions that may accompany empathy. Traditional understandings of empathy or compassion (or "pity," the term used in earlier translations of ancient philosophical texts, but now disfavored as signifying a measure of condescension) hold that a crucial component of the connection we feel with the other person through empathy comes from the realization that we are similarly vulnerable to the misfortune that has befallen the other person. It *could* happen to us. Philosopher Martha Nussbaum calls this the "judgment of similar possibilities."[3]

On the surface, this realization of our common vulnerability as human beings might appear consistent with welcome's recognition of the common humanity of all human beings (see Pattern 9). But there are important differences here. With welcome, the call to appreciate and value our common humanity has to do with understanding all humans as members of a moral community within which we owe one another obligations of care and respect. With empathy, the recognition of our common vulnerability moves in a different direction, one that again refers back to the self; we consider how the other person's vulnerability is like our vulnerability. That is, empathy makes us aware of our own vulnerability, and the emotion that often accompanies such awareness is fear, the fear that we could indeed suffer the same misfortunes as the one for whom we feel empathy. This fear can at times contribute (we make no claim that it always does) to our acting in ways that are distancing and unwelcoming.

Indeed, advocates for people with disabilities lay much of the blame for prejudice against people with disabilities on such fears. Paul Steven Miller was a leader in the disability rights movement and for ten years was the Commissioner of the US Equal Employment Opportunity Commission. He had the genetic condition achondroplasia, a type of dwarfism. Miller wrote that the "foremost" root of prejudice against people with disabilities "is that of fear: fear of the loss of autonomy and the 'there but for the grace of God go I' realization that disability can 'afflict' any person."[4] Such fears are often based on incorrect, even if empathetic, assumptions about what life with a disability is like.[5]

We explore further the distinctions between an ethics of welcome and an approach that relies on empathetic imagination by delving into two very different published legal opinions offered by judges in two very similar cases.[6] (It happens that one is from a trial court in England, the other from an appellate court in California, but we draw no conclusions from these origins.) Both cases involved a woman with extensive physical disabilities who sought the removal of the medical apparatus—in one case a ventilator, in the other a feeding tube—that was keeping her alive. Neither was terminally ill; each could potentially have lived many more years if medical treatment were continued. The legal outcome was essentially the same in both cases: The patient (in medical language—in legal language, the petitioner) was entitled, in the exercise of her autonomy, to have the unwanted medical treatment discontinued. Both courts had substantial precedent on which to base their decision, and the law—with which we have no significant quarrel—has remained the same in the decades since these cases were decided.

> At age 42, Ms. B[7] (the only name by which she is identified in the case) became paralyzed from the neck down after a spinal hemorrhage. While still in the hospital receiving care, she asked to be removed from the ventilator upon which her life depended. When the hospital refused, she sued.
>
> The judge who heard her case, Dame Butler-Sloss, agreed that Ms. B had the right to have the ventilator removed because she was mentally competent to make the decision for herself. The judge considered at length complex questions about Ms. B's mental capacity—for example, how one should understand prior statements by Ms. B that might reveal some ambivalence about the decision, and whether she should be first required to try a rehabilitation unit, where people frequently change their minds about the value of continued living following a catastrophic disability. In the written opinion, the judge quoted at length Ms. B's own testimony about why she wanted to die, her experiences, her values, and her faith.
>
> The judge did write briefly about imagining what Ms. B was experiencing. But she did so in the context of assessing Ms. B's mental capacity, not to opine on the wisdom of Ms. B's decision to die. The judge also explicitly acknowledged the limits of imagination and insisted that the point of reference should not be the observer but the "particular person" whose suffering is at issue.
>
> The judge noted that the health care professionals caring for Ms. B. had difficulty acceding to her request because they had become emotionally involved. "That situation was entirely understandable," the judge wrote, because they had "kept Ms. B alive and looked after her in every respect including her most intimate requirements."
>
> Finally, the judge took care to point out that her decision that Ms. B had the right and power to have the ventilator removed was not a decision that

she *would* have the ventilator removed. In a particularly memorable passage, the judge called Ms. B a "splendid person" with "great courage, strength of will and determination" and sense of humor. "I hope she will forgive me for saying, diffidently, that if she did reconsider her decision, she would have a lot to offer the community at large."

I want you here. That is what the judge—and the society for which she spoke—was saying to Ms. B. *You are welcome in this world, as you are.*

Elizabeth Bouvia was younger, only twenty-eight years old when her petition (which she had lost in a lower court) was heard by a panel of three appellate judges.[8] Their opinion described her as quadriplegic (from birth due to cerebral palsy), confined to bed, and in continual pain. They recognized that she was intelligent, had earned a college degree, had married and recently divorced, and had been pregnant but recently miscarried. At the time of her petition, she was a patient at a public hospital maintained by the County of Los Angeles. Ms. Bouvia did not actually require hospital care but a more suitable place had not been found for her. Because she was not consuming sufficient nutrients, and had earlier announced a resolve to starve herself, hospital staff had inserted a nasogastric feeding tube against her wishes.

According to legal scholar and disability rights activist Paul Longmore, there were other important details about Ms. Bouvia's life that should have been considered, and some that the court had simply gotten wrong. For example, she had lived independently as an adult for eight years (with some assistance from aides during parts of the day). She had become bedridden and hospitalized only after she became depressed and "refused to get out of bed." Longmore argues that because the professionals consulted to consider her mental status for the case did not have expertise in dealing with people with physical disabilities, they ignored the many "emotionally devastating experiences" Elizabeth Bouvia had recently encountered (including, among other things, her divorce, her miscarriage, and the death of her brother), concluding that her physical disability was the only reason she wanted to die, a decision they found "reasonable."[9]

Like the court in Ms. B's case, the court here explained that because the petitioner was mentally competent, she had the right to refuse unwanted medical treatment. The hospital would thus have to remove the feeding tube as she requested. What happened next, though, was truly appalling. The judges' opinion went to great lengths to confirm that Elizabeth Bouvia was making a rational decision to starve herself to death.

> She, as the patient, lying helplessly in bed, unable to care for herself, may consider her existence meaningless. She cannot be faulted for so concluding.
>
> Does it matter if it be 15 to 20 years, 15 to 20 months, or 15 to 20 days, if such life has been physically destroyed and its quality, dignity and purpose gone?
>
> Here, if force fed . . . [p]etitioner would have to be fed, cleaned, turned, bedded, toileted by others for 15 to 20 years! Although alert, bright, sensitive, perhaps even brave and feisty, she must lie immobile, unable to exist except through physical acts of others. Her mind and spirit may be free to take great flights but she herself is imprisoned and must lie physically helpless, subject to the ignominy, embarrassment, humiliation and dehumanizing aspects created by her helplessness.

These passages are so offensive that we might conclude that the judges were not actually exhibiting empathy here, but instead revealing biases and prejudices about people with disabilities (see Pattern 9). But both may be true. Empathy is not inherently incompatible with assumptions about "categories" or "types" of people, like people with quadriplegia. Unconscious beliefs and prejudgments are not always associated with disparaging or hateful attitudes, yet they necessarily influence how we imagine someone else's life.

Although the courts came to similar legal conclusions about what the law required, their written opinions could hardly be more different in approach and tone. In the case of Ms. B, the judge turns to *her*, to Ms. B, to understand her experience and to determine the fitting response to her request to remove the ventilator. The opinion is open, responsive, and welcoming of Ms. B, her professional caregivers, and other people living with extensive disabilities. By contrast, the panel of judges in the case of Elizabeth Bouvia were dismissive of her and other people similarly situated in determining whether to grant her request to remove her feeding tube. They appear from their opinion to have imagined how they would feel "in her shoes," if they had to live with her disabling medical conditions. Upon so imagining, they appear to have concluded they would rather be dead than be her and essentially said so.

The well-meaning rehabilitation specialist introduced at the beginning of this pattern also imagined what life was like for a patient. Before being corrected by his patient, our colleague appears to have "thematized" her.[10] That is, he saw her largely as a "theme"—a positive one, it is true, a theme of courage in the face of disability—but a theme nonetheless. That theme stood in place of, or at least overshadowed, who she was as a particular person and the particular ways in which she led her life.

In much of the right-to-die advocacy literature, legal briefs, and court opinions leading to legal rights to refuse medical treatment (and, in some states, to physician aid in hastening death), the "theme"—the most often foregrounded characteristic of the person for whom legal access to die is sought—is dependency on others for intimate functions, especially toileting. This characteristic takes on outsized importance and is explicitly taken to signify a category of people devoid of human dignity. In the two legal cases of Elizabeth Bouvia and Ms. B, the courts understood the petitioners' need for assistance with private bodily functions in starkly different ways. In Ms. Bouvia's case, this dependency was defining—it was her theme—and equated with a life of such poor quality that it was hardly worth living. In contrast, in Ms. B's case, the judge mentioned this dependency not as a character trait that defined Ms. B in any way but as something that had brought her and her health care providers into such a close relationship of care that it was difficult for her caregivers to accede to her request to die.

Both decisions are based on the competency of the petitioners to refuse medical treatment. *Was* Elizabeth Bouvia competent to make the decision to remove her feeding tube? We do not pretend to know. But we are troubled that the court did not require further investigation into the circumstances that brought her to this point. Paul Longmore and others have questioned whether enough effort had been made to assist her in finding a place to live and accessing other resources to which she was legally entitled but which she was not receiving. The court matter-of-factly accepted that recent efforts to find Ms. Bouvia an apartment with appropriate live-in assistance had been unsuccessful, resulting in her residency in the public hospital, which "was required to accept her." The judges did not question whether Elizabeth Bouvia's wish to die had something to do with the fact that she had nowhere to live, that there appeared to be no place in the world for her at all, or whether she was cared for, liked, or respected by anyone who was responsible for her physical care or, for that matter, by anyone at all. In contrast with the opinion in Ms. B's case, the court's opinion in Elizabeth Bouvia's case did not inquire into the quality of the relationships she experienced at the hospital with her physicians and other staff, noting only their concerns about legal liability or violating medical ethics if they ceded to her wishes.

Reading the judges' descriptions of Elizabeth Bouvia's life as having no purpose, meaning, or dignity, it is impossible to avoid the strong suspicion that they were imagining themselves in her position. They could not fathom that they—highly successful, able-bodied people—would want to continue living were they in her condition, nor could they see how anyone possibly would. Whether their conclusions were wrapped up in discomfort or fear that a similar fate could befall them is conjecture, but the emotional valence of their language indicates that this may have been the case.

The judges did move; they did act in response to whatever feelings they had when they imagined themselves in Ms. Bouvia's shoes. She was not ignored or turned away. We might even say they moved toward her; they were, after all, doing what she asked and what they believed to be in her best interests. But they *did not welcome her*. They did not want her here. At best, they were indifferent to her continued presence in the world; at worst, they preferred she were gone.

We don't want to leave the impression that there is nothing good about empathy. The motives underlying empathetic impulses are generally good, and at times imagining how someone else lives is the best we can do (see Pattern 15). But we do believe empathy must be exercised with caution and mediated with welcome. If we want to be welcoming, we need to take care that when we feel empathy, we do not presume that we know more than we do. A presumptuous empathy may lead us to think poorly of another person's choices, capacities, or presence with us. In addition, we must guard against reacting to another's presence in ways that keep them at a remove because of the discomfort that may accompany our own empathetic feelings.

Rely less on your imagination of what other persons might be experiencing. Instead, find out what their life is like from them or those close to them, if possible.

Notes

1 Martha Nussbaum writes that "compassion, in the philosophical tradition, is a central bridge between the individual and the community." Martha C. Nussbaum, "Compassion: The Basic Social Emotion," *Social Philosophy and Policy* 13, no. 1 (1996): 27–58, at 27.
2 Mohrmann, *Attending Children*, 156-7. Chapter 12 of *Attending Children* is a story about "presumptuous empathy."
3 Nussbaum, "Compassion," 34.
4 Paul Steven Miller, Esq., "The Impact of Assisted Suicide on Persons with Disabilities. Is It A Right Without Freedom?" *Issues in Law & Medicine* 9 (1993): 47–62, at 53.
5 Miller, "The Impact of Assisted Suicide."
6 These two cases are subject to further examination in Lois Shepherd, "Face to Face: A Call for Radical Responsibility in Place of Compassion," *St. John's Law Review* 77 (2003): 445.
7 Ms. B v. An NHS Hospital Trust [2002] 2 All E.R. 449.
8 Bouvia v. Superior Court, 179 Cal. App. 3d 1127 (1986).

9 Paul K. Longmore, "Elizabeth Bouvia, Assisted Suicide and Social Prejudice," *Issues in Law & Medicine* 3 (1987): 141 at 156–8.
10 We have found Levinas' work helpful here. See Emmanuel Levinas, *Otherwise than Being: Or Beyond Essence* (Duquesne University Press, Pittsburgh, 1998), 6, 153, and Adriaan Peperzak, *To the Other: An Introduction to the Philosophy of Emmanuel Levinas* (Purdue University Press, West Lafayette, IN, 2005), 97–109.

13

Everything about a Person Matters

Seeing the other person as they are, a distinctive and whole individual, is an act of respect and an essential component of welcome. It requires that we break through deeply ingrained tendencies to stereotype.

After one of us presented a talk about welcome to a large group of hospital chaplains and other health professionals, a nurse stood up to ask a question. She began by describing a patient she was currently caring for in the hospital. Her patient weighed over 600 pounds and had cellulitis—"his own fault," she added (cellulitis, a serious skin infection, is a known hazard of massive obesity). She said that she has back trouble, and the audience groaned in sympathy. Then she asked her sincere, poignant question: "How *can* I welcome this patient?" The anguish in her voice was unmistakable. Even while conveying her aversion to her patient—she described him only by his weight, blamed him for his illness, saw him as a threat to her own health—she also expressed her genuine desire to carry out her vocational and personal obligations to him, somehow.

Part of a reply to her question should surely include serious recognition of the hospital's responsibility to help her out, to provide sufficient support staff and promote an institutional culture that encourages calling for support when needed, so that she would not risk further damage to her back by trying to help her patient in and out of bed (see Pattern 28 on sharing responsibility and Pattern 29 on institutional responsibilities). But that would help only her back; it would not address the deeper issue, the aversions that effectively thwart her stated desire to welcome him (see Pattern 26 for a fuller discussion of aversions).

The nurse's question could have been asked about other kinds of patients encountered in healthcare practice. For example, a nurse could have said that he works in an emergency department where virtually every day he faces one or more members of a set of patients, by now quite familiar to him, who come in intermittently but frequently with complaints of intractable pain, clearly suffering and clearly seeking opioids. The ED is a busy one; he believes these patients take him away from others whose health problems are not "their own fault" and are likely treatable. He wants to be the ideal nurse whose image drew him into nursing and still informs his work, but how can he welcome these "drug-seekers"?

The question could also have been asked about another sort of patient encounter—although the questioner would probably have been a doctor, not a nurse. The physician, a hospitalist a few years out of residency, says that it's not unusual for her to be responsible for the care of a patient who is dying. She knows her obligations in the situation, but she's also aware of her resistance, her tenacious unwillingness to go see that patient because, she believes, there's not a thing she can do for him; she has no further role. She finds it so difficult being continually confronted by her impotence in the face of his disease that she doesn't understand how she can possibly welcome him.

This is the trap set for us by categorizing, stereotyping others. The nurse who asked the initial question, according to her presentation of her dilemma, saw her patient only as someone who was very obese and, as a result, directly responsible for the infection that landed him in her lap, so to speak. Likewise, in the hypothetical versions of that question, the nurse and doctor recognize their patients as a certain *type* of person—someone seeking drugs, someone dying—but see little more than that designation. In each of the three situations, they can find no opening for welcome because they have not opened themselves to the unique person who is their patient.

"Stereotype" was coined in the eighteenth century to name both the process and the result of printing from a solid, unchanging block of type, a three-dimensional block that can produce the same two-dimensional image over and over again. Andy Warhol's repetitive block prints of Marilyn Monroe are classic stereotypes. When we stereotype someone we encounter, then, we are seeing only the same two-dimensional "person" over and over again—another massively obese, self-negligent man; another manipulative addict. We see only the flat, impersonal image produced by our own solid mental block of type, not the actual person before us.

How *can* we welcome someone who remains to us nothing more than a 2-D stereotype? We cannot. Welcome requires that we step around and beyond the stereotype, the category that we have hastily assigned.

It may take long years of practice to break ourselves of the habit of stereotyping persons upon our first encounters with them, but in the meantime, it will help to remember that stereotyping is not in itself the primary problem. To reiterate a point made about recognition of humanness (Pattern 10): the problem is stopping there. We don't have to chastise ourselves for stereotyping but rather train ourselves, by practice, to *notice* our hasty classifications for what they are and then *move on* to open ourselves to, and thus begin to know, the individual before us. One side benefit of this practice is that it is likely, over time, to reduce our tendency to stereotype others in the first place.

In order to break through stereotypes, we must do what Count Rostov says we must (see Pattern 2): *Reconsider* this person, and then reconsider them again, and again, because every human being is too complex and too idiosyncratic to be encompassed by any superficial type we may assign them. Each of us is so much more than what we may appear to be at first glance. We are embodied, but more than our visible bodies and their distinguishing characteristics. We are rational beings, but more than our calculating minds. We are spiritual to one degree or another, but more than our enfleshed souls. The whole—our wholeness—is greater than the sum of the parts.

We often talk about ourselves and other persons as though we were divisible into "parts": body, mind, spirit. This way of speaking can be very useful for communication between and reasoning about persons, much as our division of time into hours and minutes is a very useful practice. In fact, it's hard to imagine how we'd get along without either convention. Nevertheless, we know that time is not really segmented, any more than a flowing stream is, and neither are persons. Each of us is a single unity, a whole person, with entirely integrated and interdependent bodies and minds and spirits.

We are not body plus mind plus spirit, somehow held together in this life like the interlocking pieces of a jigsaw puzzle, forming an easily fragmented entity that only appears to be a single thing. We are bodymindspirit, all in one; we are integrated, whole. This is one of the basic meanings of *integrity*: the innate *oneness* of each human being, like the oneness of an integer, a single whole number, not multiple and not fractionated.

The welcoming person sees others as whole persons and welcomes them as they are. The nurse in the story that opens this pattern does not have to welcome her patient's obesity; she is called to welcome *him*. To do so, she has to open herself to knowing him as he is, and who he is is more than his body weight or his skin infection or even, were this to be the case, his grumpy personality. We do not have to welcome the afflictions or the suffering of the persons we encounter. We have to welcome persons as they are—weighing 600 pounds, begging for narcotic relief, leaving us behind as they die, and always more than any of these typological characteristics. *Everything* about a person matters.

Welcome does not ask us to pretend that what we react to on first glance is not true; it asks us to go further, to look and think again. The nurse who asked that difficult question does not have to behave as though her back is fine and her patient really isn't very obese. Rather, she can take a second look and see that an obese body is not all he is, and an aching back is not all she is. Nor must the nurse in the ED act as though his patient is not really addicted, and he doesn't have complicated, ethically and legally fraught decisions to make. Instead, he can think again and recognize that there's more to this person than her drug craving, and more in himself than fatigue and frustration and self-righteousness. The hospitalist physician need not pretend that her patient is going to recover and that she doesn't feel helpless and afraid, but she can also see that the person who is dying is still alive and whole and that she has deep vocational skills of caring attention that are precisely what is needed at this moment.

Welcome asks that we—these healthcare professionals, as well as all of us who wish to be welcoming—acknowledge the reality of the situation, recognize and set aside our immediate reactions to the stereotypes our minds conjure up, and fulfill our responsibility to respect both the whole person before us *and* the whole persons we are.

Step beyond the temptation to stereotype others. Reconsider them, again and again.

Part III

Things We Can Do

In Part III, we consider fundamental practices of welcome—ways we can pay attention, actions we can take, things we can do—that sharpen and expand upon the fundamental perspectives of welcome discussed in Part II.

14

Practice, Practice, Practice

Becoming a welcoming person doesn't happen automatically, just because we wish it to be so. Rather, we have to practice welcoming behaviors and allow the practice itself, and what we learn from others' responses to us, to shape us into the welcoming persons we desire to be.

Several years ago, Lois' mother, Carolyn, suffered a concussion and then a series of small strokes. She was treated at an acute rehabilitation facility for a few months, during which time she had difficulty moving and clearly exhibited diminished mental faculties. She was fully awake and able to see and hear, but could feed herself only with help and respond only sparingly in conversation. Later, after her condition had improved substantially and she returned home, she said she remembered nothing about her stay in the rehab facility.

But Lois remembers it well, and she remembers one day in particular. She had driven six hours to see Carolyn, as she had been doing every week or so since this sudden and unexpected change in her mother's health. The concussion and mini-strokes had not yet been diagnosed; the fall that precipitated those events had happened months earlier, its effects unfolding only over time. So, the family did not know what was going on—which added to their distress—and they were preparing themselves for their mother's further decline and impending death. Carolyn was 83 at the time, but a few months before she had been regularly driving, teaching Sunday School, volunteering—a healthy and active older adult before this mysterious and abrupt malady.

On this particular visit, Lois, sitting alone with her rather glassy-eyed mother, could not hold back quiet tears. She was not sure that her mother had recognized her when she came into the room; Carolyn had said something general like, "How are you?" when Lois greeted her. Now, wiping away the tears, Lois said, "I'm sorry. I don't know why I'm crying." Her mother's response was, for Lois, unforgettable. Carolyn said slowly, somehow gently, although with little affect, "Well, you've been through a lot."

What? Say that again? *Who* has been through a lot?

Carolyn's reply was the response of a person who had practiced an ethics of welcome over a lifetime. She had this response in her pocket, ready to take out. She said it effortlessly, almost as if by rote, but not at all remotely. She may not have known who was sitting with her or why that person was crying, but she knew to say something that expressed kindness and concern—and she had words ready to say.

We do not intend to offer Carolyn, or anyone else for that matter, as a perfect model of welcome for all times and situations. Instead, we present this story as a depiction of what can result from having formed the *habit* of being a welcoming person.

Ancient philosophers—Aristotle, among others—characterized virtues like justice, courage, and self-control as settled dispositions to think, choose, and act in ways that foster human flourishing, individually and communally. Such habitual ways of being require both practical knowledge and a fixed intention. Justice, for one example, can be briefly defined as a set of circumstances in which each person receives their due. The just person knows how to understand what is due to whom and has an unwavering intention to see that it happens—not occasionally or incidentally, but always and deliberately. Just persons *reliably and intentionally* think, choose, and act in just ways.

This book is about becoming welcoming people, about developing the habit, the settled disposition of being welcoming. We can, therefore, describe being welcoming much as virtue ethicists describe being just or courageous: The welcoming person knows how to be open and appropriately responsive to others and has a firm willingness to do so. Welcoming persons *reliably and intentionally* think, choose, and act in welcoming ways.

The ancient teachers of virtue also admitted that they knew few, if any, people who were perfectly virtuous, displaying all the virtues all the time. Their teachings were instead about how one might come closer to that ideal, growing more aware and more adept at being just, courageous, temperate, and wise. Aristotle famously taught that, if you want to become a virtuous person, you must *practice*. To become a just person to your core, for instance, you have to consistently hone your skills of perception and deliberation in order to know where justice lies, and then consistently decide and act justly. With practice, you become able to spot a temptation to be unjust long before you're trapped in it, and the mere prospect of being unjust comes to feel so against the grain that it is unbearably uncomfortable, impossibly difficult. If you were to decide or act unjustly, you would be keenly aware in that moment of being incongruent, not whole, not a person of integrity.

So it is with welcome. If we engage in welcoming behaviors consistently and intentionally, then those approaches and actions become easier to summon, more quickly recognized and chosen. This is true even at times when we are just "going through the motions" because the inner welcoming impulse is dim or absent: it is still effective practice. Over time, our willingness to welcome others becomes more firmly fixed, embedded, such that welcome is our first and sustained approach to the people we meet—for the first time or the thousandth time—and we have become welcoming persons.

Go through the Motions

In everyday language, we tend to use the expression "going through the motions" negatively: someone's heart is just not in what they're doing, whatever that may be. A competitive swimmer does not bring their "A game" to the swim meet. A person pays "lip service" to a cause or project they do not believe in or may be secretly working to undermine.

In contrast, we present "going through the motions" as a positive activity, as a way of developing a welcoming disposition. As it happens, the phrase ties in well not only with the metaphor of dance that we have adopted as one way of understanding the method of this book but also with our insistence that moving in some way—*acting*, another word that can mean "going through the motions"—is an essential facet of welcome (see Pattern 3).

Throughout the book, we present various attentive behaviors that one might adopt—and practice until they become habitual—in order to welcome others:

Take a step toward the other person—a literal step, like entering a room, or a virtual step, like asking an attentive question (Pattern 4). Use the language people prefer for themselves, their affiliations and relationships (Pattern 16). Call people by their names (Pattern 17). Doing these things consistently—even when it does feel like just going through the motions or, to use another common expression, like "faking it"—can form in us good habits of mind, body, and spirit that deepen our capacities for perception and response and nurture our intention, our steady willingness to be welcoming people.

Sometimes we "fake it" because we don't know how, as a practical matter, to respond to the people and the situation before us. We don't have the words. We don't know whether a handshake is appropriate or a hug, or whether eye contact, usually okay, even required, in this particular instance would be intrusive. What did the Ritchies (the couple introduced in Pattern 1) do the first time they looked out their window and saw someone preparing to jump from that cliff? It's likely that they didn't know what to do—or so we imagine because we doubt we would know. But even if they wondered *how* to act, they seem not to have asked themselves *whether* they should act. The news story about them indicates that they were already open to seeing the hurting people who came to the cliff, seeing them as they were and as persons to whom they had to respond. Don Ritchie told the CBS reporter, "You can't just sit there and watch them. You gotta try and save them. It's pretty simple."[1]

But how? How to know what to do? The news feature does not recount the first incident, but it does tell us what Mr. Ritchie habitually did during the following 50 years for more than 500 individuals who stood at the edge of the cliff: He hurried over to them, smiled warmly, asked if they'd like to talk, and invited them for a cup of tea. Perhaps that's what he did the first time, too, following already developed habits of conventional hospitality. And perhaps the offer was taken up in a way that signaled to him that it was a helpful thing to do. However it came about, his thoughtfully practiced approach clearly became part of him, deepening his awareness of the people he approached, anchoring his intention to respond to them, and enabling him to go out on the cliff again and again to offer his welcome to yet another desperate person.

We're all familiar with this kind of learning. Most of us have developed, step by careful step, both the specific proficiencies needed for our work careers[2] and the communication and relational skills essential for living well with other human beings. If we are fortunate, we have had teachers, mentors, and models all along the way who have coached us into mature competence.

Medical students, for example, when they are first encountering patients, are often given relatively formulaic ways of introducing themselves, of putting the patient and themselves at ease. Their teachers suggest things to say to get them into the room and other things to say to help steer the interview around to difficult topics, so they'll be able to ask about things like drug use and sexual practices in ways that can enable an honest and inoffensive conversation about such intimate matters.

Some mentors refer to these phrases as "words in your pocket," a helpful metaphor. It's reassuring to know that something to say is stored nearby, at the ready, to be taken out when one is distracted or anxious or afraid, at a loss for words. Still, some medical students we have taught initially chafed at using introductory formulas, as well as at practicing their approaches with people who pretend to be patients for educational purposes. The students would say something to indicate they knew how to have a conversation because they had been having them all their lives. Then we'd get to the part about taking sexual histories, and all of a sudden they were less certain of their skills, for these were clearly not the conversations they'd been having all their lives. Nobody is born knowing how to do these things, especially in situations loaded with performance anxiety. So, their teachers give them things to say and ways to say them—and with time, practice, and experience, the students rewrite the scripts in their own words, now having developed the good habit of having their own words in their pockets.

When students use the formulas they've been given with real patients, are they faking it? Yes. Is that a problem? We don't think so. We all start out by faking it. Children are taught to say "No, thank you" and "Yes, please" and "Excuse me" and "Sorry"—and they say these things, but quite a bit of the time they're faking it. That doesn't make the rote repetition meaningless. Rather, these words and phrases are useful tools that they are growing into; perhaps better put, they're valuable modes of relating that are *growing into them*. At some point (at least this is the hope), they will say them or something like them habitually because they will have learned, by practice, that courtesy is a deeply meaningful expression of mutual respect and even love. They will have become courteous persons, by practice.

Lois remembers being taught by her mother to say at the dinner table of her grandmother or any host, "May I please be excused? That was delicious." She learned these specific words from a very early age; they were given to her, and she heard her older sisters say them. It wasn't until she was in her early teens that it occurred to her how odd and maybe a bit ridiculous it may have seemed that each of the four siblings, in turn, said the same rush of words as soon as it appeared reasonably acceptable to ask permission to leave the table. She began trying out variations: "The pie was delicious," "The meal was wonderful." It seems curiously funny to her even now—but even now she routinely compliments the host for the meal she's been given.

Of course, the child analogy is not a perfect one. Children initially say the words they're given not because they want to get better at being courteous, but because they've been told to do so, and they want their parents' and other adults' approval. Sometimes they even seem ironically aware that they are going through the motions. At Margaret's less formal dinner table, her grandchildren engaged in a certain amount of eye-rolling and flagrant fakery, and they seemed to think that saying "Excuse me" magically made burping at the dinner table okay.

But when we, as mature or maturing people, fake it in order to practice being welcoming—that is, when we pretend a readiness to welcome we have not yet achieved, a welcome we may not yet feel—it is nevertheless our own intentional behavior. We're choosing to behave that way because we believe we should, and we believe it's helping us become the people we want to be: people who are so habituated into a welcoming disposition that, like the Ritchies, we can look and be moved and act without having to stop and think about whether this person is worthy of our efforts or about what we may or may not have to gain or to risk by responding.

Let the Motions Go through You

An ethics of welcome clearly requires of us more than welcoming gestures. Going through the motions can only be a *start*. We also have to *let the motions go through us* so that we may experience that essential internal movement or shift described in Pattern 1: the emotional, cognitive, spiritual, physical opening and extending of ourselves toward the one we welcome now *and* toward the ones we will welcome in the future.

Ancient philosophers who taught their students about the acquisition of virtuous dispositions knew well that it is possible to become adept at a *semblance* of virtue without actually becoming virtuous. Just so, there is the risk that, with practice, we can become quite good at the *motions* of welcome without becoming someone who consistently desires the presence and well-being of the other person. On the other hand, fortunately, the ways in which we signal to another person that we desire their presence are also ways in which, if we are willing to be changed by those we meet, we can acquire or confirm or deepen that desire.

How is it that our welcoming motions can kindle in us a true desire to be with this particular person? In the first, defining patterns of this book, we declare that "I welcome you" *means* "I want you to be here." But, of course, it may be that, at times, our saying and enacting "I welcome you" may actually mean something more like "I intend to be a welcoming person," with "you" not yet in the equation. We may step toward someone in welcome without having any formed or even nascent sense of sincerely desiring the presence of *this* person. It is the work of welcome itself—opening ourselves, paying attention, seeking fitting responses, employing the perspectives of Part II and the practices of Part III—that can, if we allow it, awaken or strengthen in us the desire to be in the presence of this person we are now coming to know.

The welcoming gestures we practice may initially be pro forma, but when we also, at the same time, open ourselves—even minimally, hesitantly—to the reality of the other person and are intentionally mindful of the shared space we inhabit together—even momentarily—we cannot help but be affected by the other's presence. We are no longer quite the person we were before. As Levinas taught us, when we openly encounter another person, we experience a *rupture*, a seismic shift.³ With the right intention, the intention to be welcoming, that rupture, that breaking open, can move us from what may have been simply a sort of generic benevolence (or indifference, or even disapproval) toward a sincere desire for the presence of this person with us and in the world.

Paying attention as we practice is key, noticing how it *feels* to be open, where it leads, what prejudices have to be set aside, how we are discerning our responses and how they are received. Thus can we be shaped, changed by our encounters.

More broadly, our willingness to change, to let our welcoming motions move through us, enables us to come closer to being the consistently welcoming persons we want to be and to living as persons of integrity. After all, a defining quality of integrity—the moral art of being one person, not duplicitous, not two-faced—is congruence between feeling and doing, between internal commitment and external behavior. One way this is attained is by allowing our practiced signs of openness to others (the smile, eye contact, attentive listening, and so forth) to develop from studied gestures into effective means of awakening us to the reality of the other person.

We're Always Practicing Something

When the perennial question arises of whether medical students can learn (can be taught) empathy in medical school, one honest reply is to point to the evidence that they do learn (are taught) empathy's opposite. A medical student writes about what he observed in the hospital:

> The way we talk about patients in the workroom matters. I often catch myself subconsciously judging patients based on how others talk about them and realize that this affects the quality of care they receive. When patients are described as lazy, difficult, arrogant, or by some other insult, I believe they get a different kind of health care, at least in the way they are treated by the team. . . .

The blasé attitude some people portray is especially concerning to me as I watch classmates adopt that frame of mind. When one is surrounded by students all day, biases are contagious. We watch and we copy everything.[4]

Each time doctors or medical students walk into a room to meet a patient, and each time they then talk with others about that patient, they are practicing something. *Each time* any of us—whatever our profession or employment status, age or interests—speaks to or about a boss, an office assistant, a team member, a housekeeper in the hall, a spouse or family member at the dinner table, a contact on social media, a cashier or a customer at the grocery store, we are practicing something. *Each time* we are *either* practicing the skills of welcome, of paying attention and being open and responsive, *or* we are practicing the skills of welcome's opposite, skills of inattention, distance, and dismissal.

We are always forming ourselves one way or another. There is no neutral ground. If we are not training ourselves to be welcoming, then we are training ourselves not to be welcoming.

Being welcoming toward everyone all the time seems an impossible task, and so it may be. Welcome is an aspirational ideal. It is likely that none of us can be truly welcoming all the time, in every situation. Therefore, the point is not to judge ourselves or others for our inevitable failures of welcome but to recognize ways in which we can learn, change, do better next time, come a bit closer to approximating the ideal. This, too, is part of the practice of welcome.

The realization that we will probably never be perfectly welcoming is no reason not to try to be better at it. The stakes are too high, in all our moral interactions, to let ourselves off the hook with a facile claim that it's too much to ask. As Mary Chapin Carpenter's poignant song reminds us, it may be more than can be expected, but "Not Too Much To Ask."[5]

Practice all the possible ways of expressing your welcome to others. Practice and practice and practice.

Notes

1. https://www.cbsnews.com/news/australian-angel-saves-lives-at-suicide-spot/
2. This process is memorably presented in Patricia Benner's award-winning book about the formation of the "expert nurse." Patricia Benner, *From Novice to Expert: Excellence and Power in Clinical Nursing Practice* (Prentice Hall, 1984, 2001).
3. See Peperzak, *To the Other*, 20. In describing this phenomenon, Peperzak writes, "The other's face (i.e., any other's facing me) or the other's speech (i.e., any other's speaking to me) interrupts and disturbs the order of my ego's world; it makes a hole in it by disarraying my arrangements without ever permitting me to restore the previous order."
4. From an anonymized medical student essay.
5. The song "Not Too Much to Ask," written by Carpenter and Joe Diffie, was released in 1992. Lyrics can be found at https://www.azlyrics.com/lyrics/marychapincarpenter/nottoomuchtoask.html.

15

Reconsider, Again and Again

There are many ways to reconsider the person we welcome, to break away from the generic categories we are tempted to assign.

Setting aside stereotypes (see Pattern 13) is primarily a matter of taking another, more attentive, more open look at the person we are welcoming. We can invite them to tell us who they are, find pleasant associations, change the story we write about them in our heads.

Be Curious

Gentle, attentive curiosity is what's in play when we engage a stranger at the backyard barbecue (Pattern 5). It is a practice that can be cultivated, not as intrusive voyeurs, but as openhearted welcomers who genuinely want to know at least something about the person before us so we may respond to them as they are.

In a brief essay in the *Annals of Internal Medicine*, physician and teacher Faith Fitzgerald considered the place of curiosity in interactions between doctors and patients.[1] After pondering what might distinguish medical students perceived by patients to be kind and humane from those regarded as arrogant and distant, she asked: "What is kindness, as perceived by patients? Perhaps it is curiosity: 'How are you? Who are you? . . . Tell me more. . . . ' And patients say . . . 'She really seemed to care about what was going on with me.' Is curiosity the same, in some cases, as caring?"

She then offered an example showing where curiosity can lead. During hospital rounds, "determined to teach the housestaff that there were no uninteresting patients," she asked a resident about the patient he considered the dullest of them all:

> He chose an old woman admitted out of compassion because she had been evicted from her apartment and had nowhere else to go. She had no real medical history but was simply suffering from the depredations of antiquity and abandonment. I led the protesting group of housestaff to her bedside. She was monosyllabic in her responses and gave a history of no substantive content. Nothing, it seemed, had ever really happened to her.

But then Dr. Fitzgerald asked the patient how long she had lived in the city, the start of a string of curious questions:

> Where did she come from? Ireland. When did she come? 1912. Had she ever been to a hospital before? Once. How did that happen? Well, she had broken her arm. How had she broken her arm? . . . The boat lurched. The boat? The boat that was carrying her to America. Why did the boat lurch? It hit the iceberg.

The most uninteresting patient on the ward that day had been a passenger on the Titanic.

Just so, gentle and respectful inquiries that signal our interest in coming to know another person can effectively move us past stereotypical assumptions. "Have you always lived in this city?" One curious question often leads naturally to another, uncovering more about relationships and activities, more about this unique and complex person, until we find ourselves genuinely drawn to the story and thus to the person. Not incidentally, we may also find that any stereotype-based preconceptions we may have harbored—about who this person is or about our own inability to welcome them—are, if not entirely illusory, drastically inadequate to describe or explain either the other person or ourselves in this encounter.

Some readers may immediately raise the objection that there just isn't sufficient time to have these sorts of exchanges. Time allotment is undoubtedly an issue, but the specific question of whether there is enough time to try to know another person beyond a first-impression category has a clear answer: It doesn't take much time, not as much time as many assume (or fear). Getting to know the person before us a bit better, enough to get beyond the stereotype to the actual whole person, is not primarily a matter of time; it's a matter of willingness and preparation and practice.

Furthermore, it is time well spent. In the world of healthcare, for example, five minutes of attentive, welcoming dialogue can save hours (and dollars) expended on tests, medications, procedures, and follow-up visits that may be unnecessary, counterproductive, or harmful. There isn't enough time *not* to engage in such conversations: Tell me who you are.

Find Something to Like

Sometimes the person we want to welcome is unable or unwilling to answer our questions. This may be an emergency situation, and there really is no time for conversation. This may be a person who looks like someone we don't really want to know. In such circumstances, we can choose purposefully to regard this person in a charitable light and seek a connection by *finding something about them we like*, something that tells us of the uniqueness of this person or even reminds us of someone else for whom we have positive feelings. It could be something as simple as interesting body art or the way their hair is styled or, less superficially, some trait we have glimpsed—perhaps a certain kind of courage or determination—that we find appealing.

From interviews with healthcare practitioners recognized by their peers as "expert healers," Larry Churchill and David Schenck identified eight personal attributes and relational skills that these adept professionals appear to have in common. Among the "healing skills" was the will to "find something to like, to love" about each patient. They write, "Seeking in every patient a quality, an achievement, or even just a mannerism that can be appreciated or admired mobilizes a healing capacity in caregivers."[2] The "healing capacity" to which they refer is fundamentally an aptitude for welcome, an aptitude—relevant in all areas of life, not just healthcare—for openness toward and genuine interest in the other person that can initiate a relationship with the potential for healing, collegiality, reconciliation, friendship, and any number of other good things that nurture our lives and our communities.

Imagine a Different Story

In our discussion of empathy, we caution against relying upon our imagination to know what someone else feels or needs, rather than asking them to tell us (Pattern 12). Here, we suggest a positive, more attentive use of imagination to foster welcome.

One method of reconsidering the person before us is to turn to our own story-making abilities and *imagine*, in more or less detail, who this person might be and how they may have ended up here with us now. In truth, we do imagine such stories all the time. Stereotypes are only two-dimensional, and we tend, almost instinctively, to fill out the flat image we have conjured. Explanatory tales arise unbidden in our minds, their details reflecting our own experiences, education, and psychological leanings. Often, we don't even notice that we are creating fiction but accept our imaginings as knowledge upon which we can base judgments.

In the pediatric clinics where Margaret practiced, there was a rather common reaction by professional staff members to patients and their parents who show up at 4:30 p.m. on Friday and turn out to have nothing of any significance wrong (and thus seem not to need the clinic visit at all). The resident physicians would tell colleagues their own (imaginary) stories to explain why the visit happened and why it was outrageous, tales that often included assumptions about the child's parents being manipulative, wanting to get something free from Medicaid, or from the clinic, or from them.

But we all have choices about the stories we tell ourselves and about whether we take them to be true. These doctors—like all of us—can be encouraged to recognize that the story is their own invention, that it doesn't bear close scrutiny, and, most important, that they can choose instead to imagine a more charitable narrative, one that enables them to be more welcoming. For example, they might imagine that the child's parent returned home from work at 3:30 p.m. to find the child with minor but potentially significant symptoms. The clinic closes at 5:00 p.m. and won't reopen until 8:00 a.m. Monday. The only alternative for care, should these mild symptoms worsen over the weekend, is the emergency department. For peace of mind and best care of the child, snagging a last-minute appointment on Friday seems like the right and responsible thing to do, despite the inconveniences involved for the parent. An imaginary story like that can help the doctor approach the parent with respect, the child with professional concern and attention, and, not incidentally, be shielded from the negative effects of feeling exploited (see Pattern 21). It may even stimulate their curiosity enough to ask the parents for *their* story of why they brought their child to the clinic.[3]

Along with recognizing our tendency to categorize those we encounter, we must also be aware of the accompanying explanatory stories that arise in our minds. To truly reconsider the person we wish to welcome, we must set aside those stories and instead either elicit the truer story from the persons themselves with our curious questions or, when that doesn't seem possible, *intentionally imagine a different story, one that will enable us to be welcoming.*

Take another, more attentive and open look at the other person. Reconsider them with curiosity, generosity, and imagination.

Notes

1 Faith T. Fitzgerald, "On Being a Doctor: Curiosity," *Annals of Internal Medicine* 130, no. 1 (1999): 70–2.

2 Larry Churchill and David Schenck, "Healing Skills for Medical Practice," *Annals of Internal Medicine* 149, no. 10 (2008): 720–4, at 722.

3 We are indebted for this point to an essay by Rita Charon, which eloquently demonstrates the value of practitioners' imagining charitable stories to make some sense of troubling aspects of their patients' conditions or behaviors. See Rita Charon, "The Narrative Road to Empathy," in *Empathy and the Practice of Medicine: Beyond Pills and the Scalpel*, ed. Howard Spiro, et al. (Yale University Press, New Haven, 1993), 147–59.

16

Let People Tell You Who They Are

The best source for learning about the other person is that person.

More often than not, others tell us who they are. And, if we are open and responsive, we listen to them.

Maya Angelou famously said, "When people show you who they are, believe them" (sometimes this axiom is repeated with the addition, "the first time"). Angelou explained that if someone tells you they are "selfish" or "mean," for example, "believe them, they know themselves much more than you do."[1] She was cautioning against entering into or continuing relationships in which you ignore reliable, troubling signs at your peril. And, she says, if you undertake the relationship anyway, blame yourself, not the other person: "they *told* you who they were."

The context in which Maya Angelou was speaking was very different from ours. She was addressing a *problem* within relationships while we are focused on the *promise* of relationship. Nevertheless, we agree with the fundamental lesson: People know themselves better than we know them, and they reveal themselves, often very directly, by telling us who they are. We should listen.

But we also wish to complicate this well-known lesson with a couple of "yes, and" responses. First, however, an important stipulation: An ethics of welcome never asks anyone to enter into or remain in a toxic or dangerous relationship (nor does it offer advice about entering into romantic attachments). The essential imperative to welcome ourselves, even as we prepare to welcome others, includes understanding the personal limits and costs of welcome (see Patterns 8 and 27).

That said, an ethics of welcome also insists that we not use what another person has told or shown us about who they are as a way to force them into a flat, two-dimensional stereotype. A person who has rightly told us they are "selfish" or "mean" has not told us everything about who they are. We can both accept what the other person has said and refuse to conclude that is all there is to be said or known. Yes, and . . . ? As the previous pattern urges, welcome means that we consider, and consider again, the other person, always ready for further revelation of more and different aspects of the whole person.

As for "believe them the first time," that advice is sound as long as we understand it to mean that the person is telling us who they are *right now*, and that what is true at this moment may not be the case at another time. Human beings are constantly in the midst of change. Change is, in fact, an ethical imperative for people who welcome; when we adopt the perspectives and practices of welcome, we cannot help but change. This promise of ethical evolution is recognized in another axiom attributed to Maya Angelou: "Do the best you can until you know better. Then when you know better, do better." This option is open to all of us.

Listen to People's Stories

One common way people tell us who they are, what they need or are looking for, and what kind of response to them might be fitting, is through their stories. Indeed, in all sorts of occupations, from marriage counseling to real estate and insurance sales, practitioners are well advised to ask for and listen carefully to their client's story, the portion of their life's narrative that relates most directly to this encounter. Even in our relationships with family members and friends, we ask "What's up?" in order to invite the story of who they are today.

In health care, it has long been recognized that listening to patients' stories is an essential part of providing good care. Patients cannot be known simply through a recitation of their past medical history and chief complaint. They cannot be understood by pegging them as instances of some category (see Pattern 10) or by imagining what their lives must be like (see Pattern 12). Listening to the narrative of the situation as framed and articulated by the patient, in their own words, is essential both for appropriate diagnosis and treatment and for entering into and sustaining a relationship with them.

Lois' 82-year-old father-in-law, Marion, developed congestive heart failure. When Marion first met with his cardiologist, Dr. Achebe (not his real name) began by asking him a classically open-ended question: "Tell me what's going on." Marion began his story back in his North Carolina hometown, where he was born into poverty. He moved on to his time in the army, the back-breaking construction work he did for a living, his divorce from his first wife, and the recent death of his second wife and estrangement from his stepdaughter over estate matters. Dr. Achebe quietly listened, nodding, showing no signs of impatience.

Eventually, during an appropriate pause, the doctor asked what was going on with Marion's heart that had resulted in this visit. The conversation then shifted to descriptions of shortness of breath and swelling in his legs.

Dr. Achebe's expressions and gestures indicated that he was well aware that Marion had been telling him all along, in all the details of his life's story, what was going on with his heart. The best healthcare practitioners consistently practice this kind of respectful listening, with its carefully chosen pauses and gentle redirections, inviting the self-revelation that makes good healthcare possible. And though we have turned, as we have elsewhere in this book, to healthcare to illustrate and explicate the central importance of listening to another's story, this practice is clearly useful in all our efforts to listen well to all others.

Listen to Everything Else

There is more to listen to than the person's story.[2] Indeed, we have noticed in healthcare practices the hazards of a singular emphasis on the patient's story, not only for practitioners who have not yet developed the experience, wisdom, and patience Dr. Achebe demonstrated but also for patients less naturally inclined toward story-telling. An unnuanced focus on "getting the story" can be reductive, allowing a person only one way to communicate his or her experience of illness—through *a story*—and only one way to be known— through a story of *illness*. Not everyone comprehends life and its situations in the form of a story, with a beginning, middle, and end. Not everyone is inclined to either perceive or express their circumstances in the classic narrative format of "This happened, and then this happened."[3] Persons overwhelmed by severe pain or other forms of suffering may have no story they *can* tell, only fragmented litanies of inadequate descriptors or inarticulate laments (see the discussion of *Philoctetes* in Pattern 5).

Plus, even when there is a story to be heard, it may be related in ways that have more to do with assumptions about the listener than with the narrator's lived experience. Patients may intentionally construct a story designed to counter the one that, based on their experience of negative stereotyping and biased imaginings, they suspect their caregiver already has in mind.

In an educational film about barriers to care for persons with sickle cell disease,[4] patients describe what they experience when they try to obtain relief from pain:

> When I go to the emergency room, there's something of a stigma where they don't want to see, it seems like they don't want to see me straight away. And I see a doctor that's not willing to give me the typical medicine, the amount of medicine that will help me get out of pain.
>
> It's not even the verbal communication, it's the nonverbal communication that really gets under my skin because you get this look and you get this tone like, "Okay, you already had enough medicine, so I'm not giving you anymore." Or, "You have to have felt something." That's the worst. When I hear, "You have to have felt that," I'm like, "If I did, I wouldn't be calling, I wouldn't be bugging you every ten minutes telling you I'm in pain!"

One woman in the film explains that she is reluctant to tell a new provider the kind and amount of narcotic that has worked for her in the past because she is afraid of "being judged." The best listener on the medical staff will find it difficult to obtain an uncalculated, purely representative story from a patient who has learned the hard way to craft a tale that has the best chance of getting her what she knows she needs.

In healthcare and in every other kind of human encounter, there is always more to listen to than someone's "story." An insistence on experience being expressed as a narrative—even more so as a narrative that fits stereotypes we impose and scenarios we imagine—places serious limits on our commitment to truly *listen* to who this person is right now. The obligation of welcome insists that it is the person herself who is to be welcomed and that there is always more there than narratives can disclose. Listening to the stories others tell can give important glimpses into the whole. But there will still remain the mysterious, unrevealed core of the person, which must also be welcomed and held as it is, untold and real.

The welcoming practitioner, to return to the healthcare arena, invites, encourages, and awaits that revelation using statements or questions that are expansively open-ended and attuned to the patient: "Tell me what this is like for you." "Tell me about your pain."

Although doctors and nurses are taught to ask these sorts of questions, they often do so only as an introductory move; their welcoming stance lasts about as long as the opening handshake, as many studies have shown. Finding words that faithfully represent bodily sensations and feelings of internal disorder is not an easy task for any of us. But it is often the case that, as soon as a patient's difficulty or hesitation in replying to "Tell me about your pain" becomes evident, the nurse or doctor, in a well-intentioned effort to help and a differently intentioned effort to move things along, begins asking specifying questions. These inquiries—about location, intensity (the 1-to-10 scale), analogues (stabbing, burning), and so forth—instruct the patient that her experience has to be packaged in certain ways if it is to be comprehended and treated appropriately. She may be left feeling she has failed, has not truly represented what she is experiencing, even that she is too stupid to say it right and is wasting the busy doctor's time. Countless patients, attempting to cut through the prescribed categories in order to get their story "right," have noticed their doctor's subtle signs of irritation or waning interest and have grown silent and acquiescent.

The deeply welcoming practitioner, on the other hand, continues to wait, watch, and listen for the patient's self-revelation, allowing the time needed for the words to take shape and for the patient to be satisfied that he has indeed conveyed the truth as he knows it. There may be points at which the listener should interject brief reassurances to let the patient know she is paying attention and not becoming impatient with his halting, nonmedical vocabulary. Acknowledgment that descriptions of suffering are hard to compose and harder to deliver, recognition of a point made, and asking "Is there more?" can all be ways of continuing to welcome this person and his very own burden of pain and unease.

It is heartening to see that students entering medical school often intuitively understand the importance of waiting, watching, and appreciative listening. One of us observed a student two months into her medical education as she interviewed a patient in the hospital as a class assignment. Students were to take a medical and social history of a patient to whom they had been randomly assigned. This student, shy and somewhat introverted, spoke that day with a cantankerous elderly man with multiple medical problems. His mood alternated between bitterness and caustic humor as he threw challenging, almost needling, questions at the student while dodging most of her questions. There were awkward pauses, moments of confusion. The student pressed on. Even to an observer, the interview was uncomfortable. How was the student managing to maintain her composure so well? By the end, it had become apparent, from both her demeanor in the room and the description of the patient she related to fellow students and mentors afterward, that this student had a real appreciation for her task, which was to welcome this man and his story, however it was offered. She was more interested in getting to know him than in simply appearing to be an empathetic listener. She wanted to be in the room with him.

Pay Attention to Language

In the following pattern, we emphasize the importance of calling the person we welcome by their name—listening to the name they tell us and then using that name to address them. Some people identify themselves not only by their unique name but also by their membership in a particular set of people. Paying attention to the categories in which they choose to include themselves—an action far different from imposing stereotypical categories upon them—offers another way of understanding, respecting, and welcoming them.

One of our colleagues, Julia Taylor, is a physician who specializes in adolescent medicine. She works with teenagers who have "differences of sex development," a term used to describe conditions of reproductive or sexual anatomy that are not typical (this replaces a variety of older terms such as "intersex" and "ambiguous genitalia"). She also works with transgender youth. In a lecture to a class on Reproductive Ethics and Law, she listed many of the different labels that her patients have used to describe their gender identity—transgender, gender nonconforming, genderfluid, agender, multigender, genderqueer, third gender, and others. It can be confusing, she said. So, she asks her patients what term they use and what it means to them. She invites them to tell her how they view themselves and pays close attention to what they say. Her favorite term one of her patients uses to self-identify is "gender awesome."

In another discussion in the same class—which included graduate students in medicine, nursing, and law—medical students who were preparing to enter the field of obstetrics and gynecology explained that, in deciding whether to use the term "baby" or "fetus," they take their cues from the pregnant woman in their care. "I just listen to what the patient says, and I use that same language," one student explained. By this point in the course, the class had studied moral and legal arguments about abortion rights and learned how pregnant women have been tested for substance use or forced to undergo invasive medical procedures without their consent, as well as covered other controversial and pressing issues about which the students could and did have reasonable, even if sometimes passionate, disagreement. But when the medical students explained their use of language, the sparks of recognition in the law students' faces and the nods as they listened were striking. Here was an approach they appeared to appreciate: In the relationship between healthcare professional and patient—between lawyer and client, between friend and friend—we can use the language that the other person uses to describe his or her experience. It's not complicated.

Sometimes you hear expressions of frustration about certain groups of people wanting to be called one thing or another, about the terms changing from time to time, or about internal disagreement among members of the group about what term is acceptable or preferred. Black, African American, people of color; homosexual, gay and lesbian, queer; handicapped, disabled, person with a disability; homeless, unhoused, and so on. Sometimes this frustration is accompanied by an exasperated dismissal of the whole debate as being about "political correctness." But an ethics of welcome says: Step around that distracting argument. Listen to what *this* person, the one you're welcoming, tells you they would like to be called or how they want to be identified, and then use those words when you talk with them or about them. It's that simple.

It should also be said that an ethics of welcome does not include a role for policing others' language. When we are speaking to or about an *individual*, we are indeed obligated to use the words *that person* chooses to express their self-understanding. On the other hand, when talking about people *collectively*—for example, White people, LGBTQI+ people, differently abled people—few of us can consistently avoid making mistakes, being behind the times, or using terms different from the ones our colleagues or friends or the persons to whom we are speaking prefer. Thus, we cannot expect that people we are listening to will be able to avoid making mistakes or using terms different from the ones we prefer or believe are now current. We should take care to listen to all of what they are saying and, instead of focusing on what we might consider a language misstep, try to determine their meaning, understand their intent, and assume that their attempts to express themselves are made in good faith—and hope they do the same for us.

So much of what is discussed in this book depends upon the welcomer's willingness to listen carefully to what the other person is telling them—verbally and nonverbally—about who they are, what they think, what they are experiencing, what they need. We must listen to the other person, not to the voices in our heads that try to interpose our own needs, experiences, assumptions, and agendas. When someone tells us who they are, we should listen, and listen again. And again. When they show or tell us who they are, we should believe them *and* be open to learning more, as there is always so much more to know.

Let the person you welcome tell you—by word, cry, gesture, demeanor—what you need to know in order to form a response that fits this unique person and this one of a kind encounter.

Notes

1. https://www.oprah.com/oprahs-lifeclass/when-people-show-you-who-they-are-believe-them-video: a video of Maya Angelou and Oprah Winfrey discussing this topic, in which Angelou says, "When people show you who they are, believe them." Winfrey, later in the video, says that an adjunct to that expression, which she also learned from Angelou, is "believe them the first time."
2. In what follows, we draw on ideas previously published in Margaret E. Mohrmann and Lois Shepherd, "Ready to Listen: Why Welcome Matters," *Journal of Pain and Symptom Management* 43, no. 3 (2012): 646–50.
3. Elizabeth M. Gibson, *Encountering Narrative in Medicine* (PhD diss., University of Virginia, 2004).
4. See Carlton Haywood, Jr., "Suffering in Silence: 100 Years of Sickle Cell Disease in the U.S.," *Medical Center Hour*, University of Virginia Health Sciences Center, October 27, 2010, https://www.youtube.com/watch?v=5S3JxE_1UOw. This presentation is also discussed in Pattern 19.

17

Pay Attention to Names

Names are our deepest, most fundamental identification of ourselves. Names require care; they require that we not be careless with them.

Folksinger Jim Croce famously sang a song of himself: "Like the pine trees lining the winding road/I got a name, I got a name./Like the singing bird and the croaking toad,/I got a name, I got a name." Names form our primary identification of ourselves: I *am* [my name]. We may even mark an important transformation of identity by changing our name, or some part of it—for some of us with marriage, for example, or entry into a religious order. We alter our name in order to more accurately express an identity we've discovered in ourselves that makes our old name too childish or undignified or gender-discordant, or in order to mend a damaged identity.[1]

The ways in which we deploy names in conversation can express affection or anger, authority or submission, attention or dismissal. Most children know to pay extra close attention when a parent's commands begin with the child's full name. We pick up on the condescension evident in someone's use of our name in the middle of an exasperated statement: "I'm trying, Fred, to explain this to you," and, on the other hand, notice the powerful emotional effect of hearing our name spoken in love and affirmation: "I take you, Carmella, to be my wife."

Some aspects of our use of names reflect cultural assumptions and biases about status and value, some of them ingrained deeply enough to be barely conscious. For example, women are (still) generally more likely than men to be addressed by their first names. At a university convocation, a high-level administrator—a man who had demonstrated his commitment to gender equality many times over—introduced the six faculty members sharing the dais with him. Five of them were male, one was female, and all held doctorates and positions of equal authority and responsibility. Each of the men was presented as "Doctor [last name]"; the lone woman was introduced by her first name only. The next day, some of the administrator's staff members chided him for such blatant sexism. He denied it vigorously until shown the video recording of his introductions.

In a perhaps more conscious and surely more pernicious practice, in the American South it was long the custom for White persons of any age, including children, to assert racial superiority by addressing all adult Black persons by their first names. More, Black men were often addressed as "George" or "William," regardless of their given names.

Today, some college professors ask students to call them by their first names and confidently recommend their colleagues do the same, for the purpose of signaling that teachers and students are mutually engaged in the learning process. But many other professors, especially women and people of color, have adamantly resisted that practice. They report that they already have enough trouble getting students (and others) to recognize that they are authorities in their area of expertise and in the classroom or that they have a doctorate, are on the tenure track, hold an endowed chair, or whatever status they have earned. Far from needing to diminish their authority further, they need a practice of naming that helps them claim it.

Countless observers of medical practice have noted the not-so-subtle power play embedded in professional greetings.[2]

> One evening many years ago, on the way to the parking garage after teaching a late class, one of the authors (Margaret) tripped and fell (wearing clogs, carrying a briefcase in each hand). She smacked her head on the pavement and started bleeding from a laceration that clearly needed stitches, so she went to the Emergency Department in the medical center where she was on the faculty and regularly taught medical students about introducing themselves to patients.
>
> None of the three nurses she encountered there introduced herself. Two of them called her Margaret, first name only; the third didn't bother with a name. When the resident came in to stitch her up, he didn't introduce himself and didn't call her anything at all. As the resident prepared to suture the laceration, Margaret said, "If you're going to be sticking that needle in

my forehead, I want to know your name." He laughed and said, "I'm Doctor Edwards, Margaret," and continued his preparations.

Recognition, Connection, Respect

Names identify each of us as one of a kind, as "me" and no one else. Using them appropriately, especially at the beginning of an encounter, is not just a polite formality but a crucial moment of recognition and connection. The exchange of names is an essential part of any meaningful engagement with other persons and consequently a basic and unavoidable element of welcome. Not to offer one's name when encountering someone for the first time can rightly be taken as unwillingness or refusal to engage the other person in any but a superficial fashion. This may well be unremarkable behavior when meeting a convenience store cashier or a reasonable protection against the intrusiveness of an eager telemarketer. But it is inappropriate in an encounter in which the relationship is, or should be, anything but superficial—consulting a new attorney, meeting one's future in-laws for the first time, greeting a person who has come for medical care.

Offering one's name is a necessary early step in expressing welcome, but so is hearing and receiving the name of the other person. People who study this sort of thing tell us that the difficulty so many of us have in remembering the name of someone we've just met is not because we forget so quickly; it's because we never hear the person's name in the first place. It doesn't register. We don't pay attention. But hearing and holding, remembering, and using the name offered by the other person—or inviting it, asking for it if it's not offered—is just as important as giving our own name.

Attention to the use of names is a moral responsibility. There are interrelated ethical grounds for this obligation. For one, careful use of names is an important expression of *respect*; carelessness with names is an unmistakable sign of *dis*respect. For another, striking a balance between the names used (as opposed to the unbalanced "Hello, Margaret, I'm Doctor Edwards" approach) shows a commitment to the fundamental ethical principle of *equal regard*. It signals that I understand myself and this other person to be of *equal value*.

Sometimes, the obligation of equal regard is being honored in the face of a manifest inequality of authority or power, but an inequality of *authority* should not be mistaken for an inequality of *value*. There really isn't any way of getting around the power differential in some relationships, nor would it be a good thing if we could: Patients, for example, need something from doctors—a certain kind of knowledge, validation, access to medications or surgical procedures, and so on. The imbalance of power has even been held to be an essential ingredient in healing, at a minimum a basis for trust in the doctor or nurse.[3] Part of honoring that trust, though, is a commitment on the part of practitioners to diminish the disparities between themselves and their patients, lessening differences in knowledge, for example, by teaching and explaining. This holds true for other professions that entail similarly disparate relationships—teacher-student, lawyer-client, clergy-congregant. All such practitioners are obligated to diminish, as much as possible, perceived status differences between themselves and the people who look to them for guidance by making their respect for others as persons of equal value consistently obvious, not least through careful attention to the use of names.

The details of enacting this obligation are, as always, highly situational. We would be hard-pressed to imagine a scenario in which it would be appropriate for the doctor or nurse not to offer her or his name upon meeting a conscious patient, but whether they refer to themselves by use of their professional title or not is immaterial as long as their role is clearly defined in some way. On the other hand, if the practitioner does introduce herself or himself as "Doctor Garcia" or "Nurse Jones," then the principle of equal regard would indicate that the adult patient should be addressed in similar fashion, as "Mr./Ms./other applicable honorific [last name]," until and unless the patient requests otherwise. That does not mean that it is never appropriate to call persons by only their first name upon meeting them. At times, respect, coupled with compassion and an openness to intimate engagement, may be well expressed by use of the first name, but we caution against believing that to be uniformly or even frequently the case.

The Misuse of Names

One day on rounds, in an ICU dedicated to patients with neurological disorders, the medical team stopped outside the room of an elderly woman we will call Sarah Philips. Ms. Philips had been admitted the previous evening having suffered a stroke. After a report on her blood pressure, lab results and such, the team began to talk about what should be done next. It was clear from the discussion that the doctors assumed, because of the stroke or her age or both, that Ms. Philips did not have the ability to express her wishes about her care. But an experienced nurse on the team stepped forward to offer her observations that suggested Ms. Philips might be able to speak for herself. The attending physician disagreed and said he would demonstrate his point.

He led the group of six or seven people into the room where Sarah Philips lay sleeping. The doctor stood upright by her bed, touched her hand, and said loudly, "Good morning," to rouse her. It worked; she opened her eyes and looked around vaguely. He then asked loudly, "Is your name Sarah? . . . . If your name is Sarah, look up." Slowly she rolled her eyes upward. This seemed a good sign. The doctor looked around the room to make sure everyone saw what was happening and then turned back to the patient: "Is your name Jane?" he said. "If your name is Jane, look up." Again, she rolled her eyes upward. Satisfied, the doctor quietly told the team, "I didn't think so," and they left the room.

Playing around with anyone's name, especially the name of someone who is disoriented anyway, is wrong. The "exam" in this story is a meaningless assessment of mental acuity that does not and cannot tell the doctor what he seems to think it does (at a minimum, it is a safe bet that the doctor does not know if Jane is the patient's middle name). But beyond the problem of the test itself being pointless, the technique used is a subversion of obligations of respect and welcome. Moreover, it is a violation of the doctor's moral responsibility to act for the well-being of the patient, including not to add to her confusion and fear. Imagine what might be going through Ms. Philips' mind after this brief encounter: not only "Where am I? Who are these people? Why am I here?" but also, and more frightening, "Why don't they know my name?"

Consider another situation, more subtle and significantly more common. This particular misuse of names is often found among medical professionals who care for children. Many pediatric physicians, surgeons, and nurses at some time (some consistently so) refer to the parents of their patients as "mom" and "dad." This occurs not just when speaking *about* them, as to a colleague ("Mom is asking for an antibiotic"), but when speaking *to* them ("What questions do you have about this treatment, Mom?"). Because mothers are more likely to be the parent present at a child's medical appointments and because of gender biases alluded to above, the "mom" label is heard significantly more often than "dad."

Once again, the primary objection to addressing the parent of a patient as "mom" has to do with respect. Persons do not, upon becoming parents, lose their personhood, their individuality. They still have their own names. To address them by this single generic role title is to say, in effect, your value to me has to do only with your relation to this child, not with you as a person.

This practice is also often presumptuous. One resident physician defended his habitual use of "mom" by explaining that it is important for forming a close relationship with the parent and shows that he considers himself part of her family. But he is not part of her family, and she has not yet invited him to think of himself as such. A colleague of ours has said, wisely, that medical education is accomplished at teaching its students how to manage distance from patients but has too little to say about how to navigate closeness. The first lesson in seeking closeness, medical or otherwise, is to not assume that a relationship that needs to be mutually constructed already exists. A relationship is created by two people, not declared by one. The welcoming person signals openness to the formation of that bond, willingness to be part of it, but not assumption of immediate adoption.

To some mothers of patients, it may seem simply as though the doctor has not bothered to find out their names. Another resident explained that she prefers to call the parent "mom" because she doesn't know whether the mother and child have the same last name, and she doesn't want to make a social blunder. But the parent's name, including the last name, can almost always be found on the patient's record and, if not, there's not likely to be offense taken if "Hello, Ms. [child's last name]" is followed by some form of "Have I got your name right?" Plus, the "social blunder" of erring in a respectful attempt at getting the name right is minimal compared to the mistake of using "mom."

This problem of calling people by their generic role shows up outside of pediatrics, too. Many practitioners caring for older patients refer to them as "mom" or "dad" when discussing their situation with their adult children ("Dad may need to stay overnight"). This practice seems to entail the same problems of disrespect, presumptuous familiarity, and the appearance of not being engaged enough to know the patient's actual name, none of which can foster a family's confidence in the good intentions and competence of the nurse or doctor. It may well seem too odd to refer to the parent as "Ms. [last name]" or as "[first name]" when having a serious end-of-life discussion with her adult children, but there is still a world of difference between saying "mom" and saying "your mother."

Names matter. Many practitioners already know this and have excellent habits of practice. There is an epilogue to the story of Sarah Philips: As the team left the room, the nurse who had originally spoken up stayed behind. She bent down close to the patient's face, stroked her hair, and said, "Ms. Philips, you're in the hospital. You've had a stroke. We're going to take care of you. We've called your children."

That's what welcome looks like; that's what welcome says: I see you, I know your name, you're in the right place, here with me.

Practice getting others' names right.

Notes

1   See Hilde Lindemann Nelson, *Damaged Identities and Narrative Repair* (Cornell University Press, 2001).

2. For a relatively early, blunt, and incisive discussion of unwarranted exaggeration of the power differential between patient and physician, including "this special, intense need that physicians have to be labeled as doctors," see Samuel Gorovitz, *Doctors' Dilemmas: Moral Conflict and Medical Care* (Oxford University Press, New York, 1982), 3–22, at 8.
3. See Howard Brody, *The Healer's Power* (Yale University Press, New Haven, 1993).

18

Come as You Are

How we present ourselves and how we respond to others' reactions to our self-presentation can help or hinder the formation of welcoming relationships. It is possible to be true to ourselves and, at the same time, to be aware of how we present ourselves to others.

In a children's hospital in the early 1970s, when the Watergate scandal was at its height, an infectious disease consultant routinely wore a button on the lapel of his white coat that read, "Nixon has a staff infection." Other doctors chuckled at the pun but also noticed occasional frowns and sighs of exasperation from some parents of children he visited.

More recently, at a different hospital, a regional organ donation procurement agency distributed colorful lanyards to hospital staff, useful for displaying identification badges. The lanyards, imprinted with the name of the agency, were intended to serve as a sort of advertisement or reminder of the goodness of organ donation. Many physicians and nurses wore them daily as they interacted with patients and families, some of whom were dealing with life-threatening conditions.

How we present ourselves to others can assist or impede our intention to be welcoming. The whole of our appearance—clothes, grooming, and more—can be part of how we assure others that we are open to them and that we invite them to welcome us. Therefore, it is good practice to take care that our self-presentation does not hinder, even unwittingly, our desires to offer and receive welcome. That said, wanting to welcome others in no way requires that we suppress ourselves and our own chosen modes of self-expression. The practitioner of welcome is also invited to "come as you are."

An ethics of welcome does not mandate, or even encourage, staying within the bounds of a "conventional" appearance, whatever that may be, and certainly does not endorse judging or policing the appearance of others. Rather, it emphasizes that a sincere desire to be fully welcoming and to invite and not hamper others' welcome of us requires *attention* to how we may be perceived and, thus, to how we choose to present ourselves.

Paying attention to our self-presentation begins with our being, or becoming, *aware* that we do present ourselves in particular ways, whether or not we give it much thought from day to day. Having become aware, we can *deliberate* about our choices of dress, grooming, and display, about their significance and their purpose, considered in light of the situation and, for some of us sometimes, in the light of our vocational commitments and goals. Once our presentation is consciously chosen, we can then *anticipate* reactions we may get from those we encounter and prepare ourselves to deal well with those reactions, to *respond* in a way that fosters welcome. This is not about spending an inordinate amount of time dressing ourselves each day, but about being sufficiently aware of how and why we present ourselves, so that how others react to our choices no longer can surprise or even offend us to the point that we are rendered incapable of offering welcome. (For a clear example of the difference awareness and anticipation can make, see Pattern 8 and Margaret's story about learning to welcome herself in order to be able to welcome others as they react to her self-presentation.)

The content and weight of these recommended steps—awareness, deliberation, anticipation, response—will, of course, vary according to the particulars of the welcoming person and the role they are inhabiting. Dressing for work or for play, for a day in the clinic or a night at the opera, for an appearance in court or for the emergency department's waiting room entails different considerations of what we wish to express and the kinds of responses we hope to receive, as well as how to accommodate our own needs and preferences.

There seems little question that when one accepts the mantle of a professional—or enters into any work in which relationships of trust must be established—

one cedes some rights of free expression in order to avoid undermining the relationship from the start. Indeed, it's not easy to identify many activities in which one can be entirely free to disregard the effects of self-presentation on others. There is some kind of welcoming rationale to most occupational dress codes. When repair persons we don't know show up for an appointment at our home, it's reassuring to see the company's name on their shirt so that we know this is the electrician, not an intruder. White coats, scrubs, and ID badges let us identify healthcare workers of different sorts. Uniforms or dress codes can help establish a sort of "environmental neutrality" that is inoffensive, unremarkable, and for these reasons welcoming or, at the least, not unwelcoming.

But even in circumstances in which expectations for a particular form of dress are well established, there remain opportunities for personal expression that must be attended to with care. Clear guidelines are difficult to delineate. For example, doctors and nurses, as a rule, do not wear buttons proclaiming their political preferences, the opening anecdote notwithstanding. An often-heard message to those who would flout such conventions on the basis of self-expression is: "It's not about you; it's about the patient." But that familiar rejoinder is not always helpful or relevant, in this context or others.

Consider that medical practitioners often sport reminders of health advice and advocacy on their work clothes and can assert that such displays are, in fact, precisely for the benefit of their patients. A button showing a lit cigarette with a negating diagonal line slashed through it, or one of the ubiquitous looped ribbons supporting the fight against a particular disease, seems to be generally acceptable. But other messages may be off-putting to observers, even when the practitioner displaying them understands them to be within the realm of health promotion. Wearing a button to promote gun control or healthcare finance reform, for example, may be understood by the wearer to be an urgent matter of public health advocacy and ultimately to advance the interests of their patients generally. But an individual patient—the person with whom the practitioner desires to forge or sustain a relationship—may read it as a purely political and even infuriating sign.

A welcoming encounter—medical or otherwise—involves, at the least, two people, each of whom is allowed and should be invited to bring themselves as they are to the encounter. Rather than relying upon the admonition, "It's not about you; it's about the other person," it is truer to the meaning of welcome to say, "It's not about you; it's about the relationship." Does my self-expression threaten to impede the formation or continuation of an open connection with this person?

This question requires thoughtful deliberation. Modes of personal expression do not simply fall into one of two boxes: neutral and therefore acceptable, or provocative (in some way) and therefore unacceptable. Consider the situation involving the labeled lanyards noted at the beginning of this pattern. An observer asked a few doctors whether some patients or their families might be disconcerted by seeing their physician—the one they must trust to do everything to preserve the life and well-being of themselves or their loved ones—proclaim overtly at each visit a commitment to procuring organs for other patients. That query was met with outrage: "But organ donation is a very good thing!" Of course it is, but that doesn't answer the question about how patients and families may react to seeing that particular form of advocacy around their doctors' necks and how that reaction may interfere with forming relationships of trust.

It's easy to overlook ways in which the clothes we don or the symbols we wear can unintentionally push others away and impede our efforts to offer and sustain welcome. Awareness and deliberation are key: Is this mode of self-expression I have chosen—this article of clothing, hairstyle, body art, political button—important enough to me and my sense of self that I am willing to risk that someone else might find it a barrier to welcome? Am I willing to do the work needed to try to overcome that resistance?

As one example, some people routinely wear religious symbols as part of how they present themselves to the world. These sorts of insignia are part of the uniform of clergy and a form of personal expression by others. Healthcare professionals, for example, may wear jewelry or head coverings that identify them as adherents of a particular faith. An ethics of welcome does not ask anyone to avoid doing so. However, the choice to display faith-identifying symbols must come with the awareness that they may create reservations in certain patients who wonder if their being of a different faith, or no faith, could result in misunderstandings or even a lesser level of care or attention, or who may simply be disconcerted by it. In order to make welcome possible, a physician or nurse who, say, routinely wears a Christian cross must prepare herself to notice and to respond well to a patient's associating her with everything they find objectionable about Christianity.

For another example, although clothing fashions and hairstyles are certainly less strictly gendered than in the past, they remain primary cues for quick conclusions about whether someone is male or female—and many people continue to believe that everyone must be one or the other. Modes of dress, grooming, and demeanor that blur or cross conventional gender boundaries can be confusing or even repellent to people who value the clarity of the categories. That does not mean such styles should be avoided, but that the possible reactions should be anticipated and then responded to in ways that do not foreclose welcome. As with the display of religious insignia, the purpose of anticipation and preparation is to avoid our own surprise and reactive affront that can derail our most sincere desires to be welcoming.

We have moved from relatively superficial choices about dress to deeper issues of religious and gender expression. At each level, there are choices to make about the balance between self-expression and the desire not to push others away. Let us be clear that we are in no way arguing that the appropriate welcoming choice is to suppress one's inclinations and opt for some sort of conventional "neutrality," attempting to spare others even the possibility of alienation and confusion. Such a position would represent a remarkably patronizing presumption about the inflexibility and narrow-mindedness of other persons, not to mention the fact that whatever constitutes so-called conventional neutrality—a business suit and tie, perhaps, or a sweater set and pearls—is likely to be itself considered ridiculous by someone. Plus, for many of us, what some might call a "neutral" presentation is not at all neutral but self-distorting and self-destructive, a convention that would impose the *wrong* identity were one to conform to it. To be welcoming does not require any such thing of us.

Moreover, the examples offered thus far concern forms of self-presentation about which we have some choice, even if constrained. But, for all of us, there are aspects of our self-presentations about which we have no choice at all. It is literally impossible to change some identifying markers: skin color, certain facial features, a wheelchair. In regard to such immutable facets of our appearance, the welcoming person's attentive deliberation can only be directed toward anticipating and preparing to respond well to others' possible reactions. The question here is not *whether* to expose oneself to such reactions but *how* to do so, how to fulfill our obligations of welcome in such a situation, and at what cost, with what limits.

Be thoughtful about your self-presentation, anticipating and responding to others' reactions in ways that foster welcome while also remaining true to yourself.

19

Let Others Come as They Are

How others present themselves has an effect on whether and how we welcome them. Part of practicing welcome is paying attention to this influence, moving from reaction to response.

A first-year medical student, assigned to observe a community primary care practitioner, told his advisers about a patient-physician interaction he found troubling. He said that everything went well initially as the doctor, a man, explored with the patient—a shy, hesitant woman—the symptoms that had brought her to seek his help. Then, in the process of the physical examination, the doctor realized that his patient was a transgendered woman. He sprang back from her in surprise and angrily, loudly chastised her for not giving him this information from the beginning. She got up, dressed, left the room and the building, without saying another word.

This is a physician who has not thought enough about the realities of other people's lives and the ways they therefore present themselves. Nor has he given sufficient consideration to the commitments of his vocation or, for that matter, the obligations we have to each other regardless of our professional role.

Standard accounts of professional responsibility and health ethics—as well as any reasonable account of the ethics of human interactions generally—would find this doctor's reaction unacceptable. Perhaps he has convictions, religious or otherwise, about the permanence of gender assignment at birth that cause him to find her transition so offensive that he is unable to serve as her physician. Regardless, he still has a clear professional and moral obligation to treat her with respect, explain himself to her as politely as possible, and, if necessary, help her find another physician. And, under long-standing legal rules, he cannot simply abandon her.

How might a welcoming practitioner have handled the discovery of the transgendered patient's anatomy? According to the student reporter, it was a rather routine physical examination, and she had mentioned nothing about transitioning. We can well imagine that the doctor would be surprised and might have some difficulty concealing it. But a doctor intent on being welcoming would be prepared to receive and process new and unexpected information of any sort in a way that allows welcome to be sustained. For example, the doctor could respond (see Pattern 2 for the distinction between reacting and responding) in a way that is honest, direct, and caring, something like, "Oh, you're transgendered! I apologize for my surprise. I had not suspected this." Offered with a smile and reassuring eye contact, such a response could even be received as an affirmation of the patient's successful self-presentation as female. The physician might then follow up with inquiries about how the patient's transition has been, whether there have been any obstacles to care, and how the physician might be of assistance. This script isn't perfect, but we can always improve if our intention is to be welcoming.

But there's another question to ask of this story. Did this patient have a responsibility, under the demands of welcome—which apply to her as well as to the doctor—to tell him from the beginning that she is transgendered? Maybe so, if the symptoms were directly related to her genitalia or to her hormone therapy. But sometimes a rash is just a rash, arthritis just arthritis, and a layperson may not know what's relevant and what's not. Ideally, when it was clear that a physical exam would take place, she could have helped him welcome her (see Pattern 24) by saying something like, "There's another thing you need to know, because I don't want this to come as a surprise." That would have been a kind, welcoming thing to do. It also may have spared her his reaction and thus been a protective, welcoming act toward herself.

At the same time, it is asking a lot—perhaps too much—to expect a person who has undergone the social, physical, and psychological challenges of gender transformation to be boldly forthcoming before knowing how she is likely to be received. She is not obligated to disclose beyond her self-presentation as female simply in order to spare an unprepared, unprofessional physician a jolt of surprise or, in this case, apparent revulsion. In fact, his actual reaction helps us understand why she may rightly be reluctant to tell, and it makes even clearer the urgency of welcome as an essential attribute of good care—and an essential attribute of human community.

Welcome is a moral obligation incumbent on every human being, so those we desire to welcome are also obliged to be welcoming to us—and, therefore, to consider how they present themselves to us, as discussed in the previous pattern. Whether they do so or not, of course, is not under our control. We can speak directly in this book only to those who wish to be welcoming. And we do not argue, explicitly or implicitly, that a welcomer can or should try to enforce welcome's obligations on others.

However, awareness of the significance of others' choices does allow us to recognize both their effects upon us and our often unwarranted expectations and assumptions. As one unsettling example of the harm that can be done by unexamined expectations about how someone else should look or should behave, we refer again to the teaching video produced by professional staff at Johns Hopkins Medicine that we mention in Pattern 16.[1] In it, a woman with sickle cell disease explains that she carefully edits what she tells doctors and nurses about the pain of her sickling crises and the doses of narcotics she usually needs to relieve it for fear of being labeled a "drug-seeker" and receiving inadequate care as a result. She then tells what else she has learned from her many visits to the ER: In the midst of her abdominal pain crises, when only loose clothing like sweat pants is tolerable, she nevertheless dresses for the doctor as though she were going to work so that she, a Black woman in severe pain, will be taken seriously. This patient's attention to her self-presentation is grim evidence of her unfortunate past experiences with unwelcoming practitioners, and it goes well beyond what should reasonably be expected of her.

Welcome asks healing professionals to be open to and accepting of the many ways, some highly unconventional, in which persons may present themselves for care. This demand goes beyond the diagnostic importance of paying attention to a patient's affect, grooming, gait, and other important clues. There is a deeper moral responsibility: the obligation to welcome the other person *as she is*, including *as she has chosen to present herself*.

Welcome asks this openness not just of healthcare providers but of us all:

A conventionally dressed customer enters a store to browse. The person behind the counter—apparently the only staff person present at the time—is dressed in a flowing black robe dappled with rune-like figures and sports a multi-hued wig and thick, colorful makeup. It is not Halloween season nor is there any obvious connection between the clerk's attire and the goods for sale in the store. The clerk leaves the counter and approaches the customer.

What does welcome ask in this situation? The clerk bears a responsibility, including but not limited to their employer, to help the customer get past their appearance, perhaps by making light of it or mentioning an abiding interest in cosplay. The customer's responsibility is to look again and see the person, perhaps even ask curious questions. It is up to each of them to keep their differences from impeding welcome. What welcome does not countenance is the customer upbraiding the clerk or walking out in a huff, or the clerk refusing to admit or deal generously with the customer's surprise and possible discomfort.

Welcoming persons, whatever their role, are not pushed away by the merely unconventional, no matter the convention being set aside. We welcome others *as they are*.

Be thoughtful about others' self-presentation. Be open to their choices and give them the benefit of the doubt.

Note

1   See Carlton Haywood, Jr. et al., "A Systematic Review of Barriers and Interventions to Improve Appropriate Use of Therapies for Sickle Cell Disease," *Journal of the National Medical Association* 101, no. 10 (2009): 1022–33; and Haywood, Jr., "Suffering in Silence."

20

Check Your Agenda

Welcome permits no hidden agendas.

Welcome requires transparency. If our primary agenda for what appears to be a welcoming encounter is concealed, then the performance of welcome becomes something else entirely.

> A couple is at the bedside of their daughter who was severely injured in a terrible accident. She is unconscious, on life support, and may die from her injuries. The next few days will be critical. A woman enters the room to speak with them. She wears a hospital identification badge and tells them that she is there to support them in this difficult time. She spends several hours with them over the course of the next few days, offering supportive counseling. She is comforting, knowledgeable, and a good listener.
>
> During this time, the daughter's condition worsens to the point that doctors determine that she is dead by neurological criteria (commonly known as "brain death"). She is still on ventilator support to provide her body with oxygen, but specialized tests reveal that her brain has irreversibly lost all function. Once the doctors deliver this news to the parents, the woman who has been sitting with and supporting them during this time delicately turns the conversation to the issue of organ donation. It turns out that she is an employee of the regional organ procurement organization.

How should we think about this situation? There is undeniably some good that can come from practices like this. The organ procurement organization (OPO) justifies its "early family support program" ("early" because it comes before a request for organs) as a means of both increasing the number of donated organs and providing needed support to families in crisis. The program is also in keeping with both the letter and the spirit of the law. Current law requires that the families of all patients who die in a hospital under certain medical conditions be asked whether they would consent to the donation of their relative's organs; that the request follow, and never precede, a determination that the patient is dead or a decision to remove life support; and that someone specially trained to seek consent for organ donation (generally an OPO representative, not the medical staff) make the request. The roles and actions are specified in this way to reduce any conflict, or appearance of conflict, between care for the patient and efforts to procure organs for other patients. In addition, it has been shown to be helpful in a number of ways for the person who makes the request for organs to be already known to the patient's family. This, then, is the *objective* of the early family support program: to facilitate the conversation about organ donation, once that conversation is permitted, by having it take place between people who already know and trust one another. And, indeed, it has been successful. The OPO has had higher rates of organ donation since implementing the program.

Despite this success, critical care nurses who observed the program in practice expressed concern. They knew all the reasons, and the data supporting them, for considering the program a good and useful innovation. But even though it appeared to be a clear success under a utilitarian calculus, weighing overall benefits and harms to determine moral correctness, they were still uncomfortable with it. Why? Because of the OPO representatives' hidden agenda. The family support coordinators from the OPO appeared to family members to be part of the healthcare team rather than from a separate organization, much less one dealing with organ procurement. Their name tags, issued by the hospital to allow them access to clinical areas, looked like those of other hospital employees. When they introduced themselves, their affiliation with the OPO was not made clear. Even when the name of the regional OPO— an upbeat, generic name that includes the word "life"—was provided, it did not indicate the organization's purpose.

The nurses also questioned whether the OPO's stated justification for their early access to families—to help families in a time of crisis—squared with their practices. They understood the OPO's support services not being offered to families of dying patients who were medically unsuitable to be organ donors, families who would not later be contacted by the OPO. But there were other families left out as well, specifically families of patients who had previously designated themselves as organ donors on their driver's license and for whom, therefore, family consent for organ donation was not needed. These families *would* later be in conversation with the OPO representative, who would explain to them that their relative had already consented to donation and how the organ procurement would proceed. That is, these families differed from those who received "early family support" from the OPO only in this matter of consent. But they too were keeping watch, in shock and grief, at the bedside of their loved one. If the program were truly focused on family support—rather than solely on improving the odds for donation—where was the care for these families?

The basic problem is that the OPO's family support program, when conducted as described, gives the appearance of providing an uncomplicated, warm welcome in the context of a genuine caring relationship when it is, in fact, aimed at something else altogether. The counselors may be openly responsive, generous, and truly supportive to the family members with whom they interact—we would expect this to be the case—but there is no getting around the fact that the *intention* underlying their actions is to procure organs. Welcome, as we say repeatedly, is a matter of intention; when intention is focused elsewhere, welcoming actions are not genuine. (We return to this story in Pattern 29 to consider the hospital's response to the nurses' objections.)

Could we not say that nurses also have agendas all day long, as they communicate in ways calculated to achieve certain ends? For example, when a nurse enters a patient's room and cheerfully introduces himself to family members, he may be hoping to start a conversation in which he will learn information relevant to the patient's care or find out who is charged with making decisions on the patient's behalf when necessary. The nurse's disposition and words appear to be welcoming, but are they? Are the nurse's actions any different from what the OPO early family support program is doing?

It seems clear that they *are* different and that the nurse's actions, unlike those of the OPO representative, are truly welcoming. The nurse is trying to achieve certain goals through his welcoming actions, but those goals are in service of care of the patient. In contrast, the OPO coordinator's actions, even if they serve the patient's family in some manner, are designed to serve others (patients who may ultimately receive donated organs). It is this dual loyalty that the coordinators are keeping hidden. They appear to be acting solely for the benefit of the family when they are actually acting primarily for the benefit of others.

In the healthcare stories we discuss in this book, it is generally clear that healthcare practitioners' intentions in welcoming patients include not only welcome itself and the formation of some level of relationship but also accurate diagnosis and effective treatment, relief of pain, restoration of health. All of these purposes are interconnected. None is contrary to the intention to welcome, and none has to be hidden.

A multiplicity of aims is characteristic of many of our efforts to welcome others in any setting because welcome is about responding appropriately to another person, and fitting responses can take many forms. We welcome someone because, among other reasons, we sincerely want to know them, show our respect, help them in some way, ask for their help, invite and learn from their perspective, interest them in joining us on a project, and so on. Our open responsiveness to them makes it possible to see what fits and what doesn't, and each possible agenda item has the potential for deepening and extending our welcoming of each other.

Having more than one item in the agenda we bring to an encounter is not, in itself, a problem. Rather, problems arise when agenda items have to be concealed because they, and not welcome itself, are what we actually intend. That they must be concealed to be successful indicates that such hidden agendas run counter to the spirit and meaning of welcome.

Put simply, the complex agenda of welcome is to be open and respond appropriately to another person as someone of value, whether to help or to comfort, to ease their suffering, enjoy their company, advocate their cause. The agenda can never be to use, exploit, harm, take advantage of, manipulate. Welcome and its various agenda items must be integral to each other, all parts of a welcoming intention, a welcoming whole.

Examine your agenda. Be sure that each purpose is compatible with welcome.

21

Worry Less about Being Manipulated

Excessive concern that we are being manipulated—and the injury to pride associated with it—can prevent us from engaging in welcoming behaviors.

In Margaret Edson's play *W;t*, the lead character, Dr. Vivian Bearing, a professor of English literature, is dying of cancer and looks back with regret on her past lack of empathy toward her students. In a flashback scene, one of those students requests an extension on the due date for a paper. Bearing replies with sarcasm: "Don't tell me. Your grandmother died."[1]

Given the age of the average college student's grandparents, the death of one of them is a relatively common reason for a student to need time off or an extension on work due—and can also be a convincingly fabricated excuse for not having work done on time. The play's script implies that the student's grandmother had in fact died, but whether she had or not would apparently not have affected the professor's sarcastic reply. Bearing's ready cynicism meant she granted no extension and offered no words of sympathy. Her refusal to be manipulated stopped her, in that moment at least, from caring one way or the other—caring enough about a grieving student to offer kind words or caring enough about an erring or perhaps overwhelmed student to offer corrective guidance.

In the previous pattern, we discuss how an ethics of welcome insists that we "check our agenda." When we interact with someone—face-to-face, virtually, or even indirectly—we take stock of the various objectives we may have for that interaction and make sure, to the extent possible, that our pursuit of those objectives does not quash our ability to engage in genuinely welcoming actions or cause us to offer a fake welcome instead of a real one. A truly welcoming person does not exploit, take advantage of, or manipulate others.

In this pattern, we explore a corollary proposition: a truly welcoming person does not allow the knowledge or suspicion that the other person is being manipulative to interfere with their primary obligation to be open and responsive to that person. To use a sports metaphor, coming with an agenda is an "offensive" play; worrying about being manipulated is a "defensive" strategy. Neither one promotes welcome.

One of the difficult practices of welcome is learning to shrug off, to relinquish our fears of being manipulated in order to remain clear about our responsibilities and our choices. This can be quite hard to do. Sometimes it is even difficult to see that we are taking an unduly defensive posture.

> A man seriously ill with a tuberculosis infection resistant to most drugs was admitted to the hospital for treatment. Because he was highly contagious with a potentially lethal disease, he was given a private room and told firmly that he had to stay in that room in order to protect others, especially other vulnerable patients. Nevertheless, he frequently left the room, taking the elevator and wandering the halls of the hospital. When repeated persuasive efforts failed to keep him confined, the staff resorted first to taking away his clothes; he continued to wander in a hospital gown. They then had him handcuffed to his bed and, after obtaining a detention order, had a guard placed at his door.

This story is discussed in an essay about the use of "cases" in bioethics[2] as an illustration of the importance of pursuing the details, the particularities excluded from such terse accounts (see Pattern 2 for a similar point about the "case" of JR). As presented, the narrative portrays a willful, heedless patient whose cavalier actions push the staff to take necessary, if draconian, measures. However, when certain details become clear, that interpretation comes into question. The patient's room was very cold and, given a shortage of blankets, he was allowed insufficient covering for his bed. He had been promised a television and telephone in his isolation; neither one worked. No physician had spent time with him because the doctor assigned to his care was pregnant and fearful of exposure to his tuberculosis. The revised picture suggests someone left alone in a very uncomfortable room with no link to his family and friends, nothing to occupy his time, and little chance to talk about his illness and his treatment. Why should he stay in the room?

After a week or so of this turmoil, the patient was moved to a different, warmer room with a working TV and phone. His wanderings ceased, and his illness was treated. It appears that the right question (Why are you leaving your room?) had been asked early on, but the answers (It's cold; there's no TV and no phone; I never see a doctor) were not taken seriously at first. Instead, the staff quickly turned from persuasion to coercion. We could attribute the harsh actions taken to stop the patient's wandering to any number of causes, such as truly urgent concern for the health of others, including themselves, as well as troubling shortages of time and patience as well as of blankets. Perhaps various biases were in play; the patient was Hispanic and HIV-positive as a result of IV drug use. But underlying and feeding them all, we can detect staff members' resistance to being manipulated, to "catering" to the wishes of a patient who really just needs to obey the rules.

On the face of it, that last statement is ridiculous. Think of all the time, effort, risk, expense, and worry that would have been saved if he had been "catered" to and moved to the warmer room with a TV and phone as soon as possible. Plus, consider the vocational obligations of healthcare providers to attend to—not ignore or dismiss—the comfort needs of patients, regardless of their diagnoses or habits. What appears to be at work here is the tremendous, distorting, derailing power of the refusal to be manipulated.

We have surely all seen, at some time, instances in which bizarre things happen and simple solutions to conflicts are overlooked because some people have their backs up. Anticipation or fear of being manipulated can even harden into practiced ways of being. Past experiences or inappropriate stereotyping can lead us to approach someone in a defensive posture, prepared to protect ourselves from being used—as in Professor Bearing's snap answer to the student—and, consequently, unprepared to respond to what actually is happening in the encounter. Our assumptions about another person's likely behavior may not be off-base, but our concerns about being duped—especially when combined, as they so often are, with feelings of personal aggrievement or injury to pride—can cloud our judgment and close off possibilities of connection.

There is no question that some (maybe many) people are sometimes (maybe often) manipulative, seeking to exploit others for their own gains or simply not trusting that they can get what they need any other way. It is also undeniable that there's nothing to like about feeling manipulated. But the person who wants to be welcoming learns, by practice, to employ a "yes, and" approach in the face of a manipulative person (a strategy also deployed in Pattern 16). *Yes*, this person is trying to manipulate me, *and* I do not allow their efforts to deter me from being the person I want to be or from carrying out the vocational responsibilities to which I am committed.

There is nothing easy about this practice. At least most of us seem to have an almost instinctive negative reaction when we sense that someone is trying to get something from us that we think they do not deserve. We say a lot in this book about the importance for being welcoming of learning to respond rather than react, but some instincts can make a reasoned response almost impossible, and the very deep-seated fear of being taken advantage of, being played for a fool, seems to be one of them.

But, being focused on potential injury to pride, diminishment of social standing, what others might think, or even what we think of ourselves interferes with our ability to perceive situations and persons as they really are, to understand what is being asked of us. We can fail to attend to what is at stake in the encounter and be unable to clearly evaluate ethical principles that may be involved in order to discern appropriate resolutions. In a fit of pique, we may even abandon our personal and professional commitments, somehow convincing ourselves that it is morally better to tie the patient to the bed than give him more blankets and a working TV, better to sarcastically dismiss a student's request than discern what guidance is needed.

The defenses we erect to avoid being manipulated turn against us when, by refusing to agree to—or sometimes even listen to—whatever the other person wants, we allow their behavior to manipulate us into acting like a person we don't want to be. No one likes to be duped, outfoxed, blackmailed—all negative terms implying that someone else has control over our actions and decisions. But it is one thing to instinctively recognize manipulative behavior, and quite another to actually cede control of our decisions to the manipulator.

What then does an ethics of welcome ask of us when we feel we are being manipulated? First, let us be clear about what it does not ask. It does not ask us to abandon all sense of pride, to forgo our expectations of civil behavior from others, or to ignore appropriate boundaries. It does not ask us to give people whatever they want or demand, and it does not mean we cannot set limits on the fitting responses we offer within welcome (see Pattern 27). Also, and more basically, an ethics of welcome does not ask us to pretend not to notice another's hidden agenda. Being truly open to someone else in welcome means that we inevitably see attempts at manipulation for what they are. Welcome then asks that we respond appropriately, in a way that fits not only that awareness but also so much else, including the person's actual needs and our own abilities and limits. Yes, and.

It must also be said—in thinking about "our own abilities and limits"—that there are some persons who have been persistently manipulated, used, exploited, discriminated against over long stretches of time. For such persons, just recognizing the manipulation may be extraordinarily difficult, and it may be achievement enough without expecting them to fashion a robust "yes, and" response. It may be most important that they step away from such a situation, once recognized, and protect themselves. In Pattern 26, we discuss in more depth circumstances such as this one, in which someone cannot be expected to be the one to welcome some other particular person.

For those for whom being manipulated is only an occasional occurrence, we offer this antidote to the fear of being controlled that manipulation engenders: When we do recognize that someone is trying to manipulate us—by lying, wheedling, bullying, gaslighting, or whatever form it may take—we then consciously, in full awareness, *choose our own actions*. We can call out someone's lying or bullying and still be welcoming. And even if the chosen actions appear to "cater" to the other person's demands (an extension of the paper's due date, a blanket and TV), we have not, in fact, been manipulated.

We have acted on the basis of our own choice, made in full awareness of this person and of all that's going on.

Worry less about whether someone is trying to manipulate you. Learn to shrug a little more readily. Ask yourself what really matters here and now.

Notes

1. Margaret Edson, *Wit* (Dramatists Play Service, Inc., 1999), 50–1.
2. John D. Arras, "Principles and Particularity: The Role of Cases in Bioethics," *Indiana Law Journal* 69 (1994): 983.

22

Be Open to Interruptions

Routine and habitual ways of doing and thinking can be highly useful as we go about our daily activities. But they can also make us less open to being interrupted by the persons in front of us, especially those who call for unexpected responses.

A man with a debilitating neurologic disease was going through security procedures at a busy airport. He walked slowly, using a cane for support. His left hand and arm had little ability to move on their own, but his right arm could help move them into place—slowly. He had to relinquish his cane to the conveyer belt for scanning, so his progress towards the whole-body metal detector was even slower and more precarious than usual.

The Transportation Security Administration (TSA) agent on the other side of the scanner gestured to him impatiently and repeatedly barked out the order to "Step forward!" Easy for her to say. Once he got into the scanner, frazzled by hurrying, his right hand was able to lift his left arm only to shoulder height. The agent exploded, screaming "He can't raise his arm!" She called for help from other agents, then snapped, "Get back out of the scanner NOW!" As he tottered out, she continued yelling and gesturing at him to move aside so others could go through the screening.

Fortunately, another agent came forward in response to her outburst. He welcomed the passenger with words of encouragement and understanding, found him a chair to rest on, and then assisted him successfully through the scanning procedure.

There are many routines now associated with air travel and its attendant security measures. Rituals of lining up, removing shoes, being sure liquids are appropriately sized and packaged, and so on, all overseen by a busy staff of TSA agents whose primary goal is ensuring safety in the air—and whose secondary goal is keeping everyone moving through to prevent backups. Dealing with the general public at a site characteristically full of stress and impatience is not an easy job, and getting into the zone of a well-rehearsed routine can surely help things go more smoothly. Having formulaic things to say, being quick to recognize potential holdups, and politely urging people to move along are steps that assemble themselves into a protocol. But these routines can also render agents unable to see the conditions and needs of individual passengers negotiating the journey to their flights.

Sociologist Daniel Chambliss has written incisively and poignantly about the routinization that characterizes modern hospitals.[1] He describes the many ways in which daily routines and protocols, coupled with the sort of desensitization that arises from being constantly in the midst of seriously dramatic events, can blind medical professionals to the moral issues that pervade clinical situations. His insights are also applicable to the many other areas of human endeavor and interaction that lend themselves to the development of habitual practices, settled ways of doing things. Routine modes of behavior can keep us from seeing who it is and what it is that require our attention as we encounter someone.

We discuss in Pattern 14 the usefulness of having "words in our pockets," ways of introducing ourselves, initiating conversations, and responding to overtures that can ease us through the potentially awkward fumblings of a first encounter. But sometimes the words we keep in our pockets are not the right ones for the situation. For example, the person who asked Kevin Hines, the troubled young man preparing to jump from the Golden Gate Bridge (Pattern 11), to take her photo may well have approached him with the courteous words she was in the habit of using to introduce herself to a stranger, words that, in another situation, could have signaled a desire to welcome him. But she didn't pay attention to his obvious distress, an anguish that called for words outside her routine, words to match the urgency of his situation: "What's the matter? How can I help?" Sometimes our pre-scripted phrases can impede rather than facilitate welcome, especially when our reliance on those words distracts us from paying attention, from the start, to the person we're welcoming, the sort of attention that helps us learn what words, if any, are appropriate. The person before us must take precedence over our routine.

Also in Pattern 14, we briefly consider the Levinasian concept of "rupture," the surprising and sometimes unsettling change that an open encounter with another person can cause in us. When we are fixed within our reliance on the way we've always done things, it is difficult to allow that rupture to happen. But to achieve the openness welcome requires, we have to let ourselves be broken open, ruptured or interrupted by the present reality of the other person.

> A young lawyer at a corporate law firm was assigned to a case the firm had accepted pro bono from an Elder Law program. The client, a woman in her 80s, had been swindled out of her modest house. She had signed a document that she thought allowed her house to serve as collateral for loans for her granddaughter, but the document was actually a deed. She had signed over her house for loans worth less than a tenth of its value. The law firm sued the devious lender, but the lawsuit dragged on.
>
> One afternoon the lawyer got a call from the client, whom she had met only once before: Would she come with her to the Social Security office tomorrow for an appointment? It appeared that her monthly Social Security check—on which she was entirely dependent—was going to be drastically reduced because the government understood her to be receiving financial assistance from her granddaughter. That is, although the granddaughter may have thought she was making monthly "loan" payments, she was actually paying her grandmother's rent because the house was now owned by the lender.
>
> The lawyer knew nothing about Social Security regulations and had never been to a Social Security office. When she asked the firm's supervising partner what to do, he said the firm had agreed to help the client get her house back, not to help on any Social Security matters. Besides, the firm had no experience with that sort of thing. He recommended a referral to the local Legal Aid services. Legal Aid refused to take the matter because she was already the firm's client. The lawyer then tried to research Social Security issues, but quickly determined it would be impossible to prepare for the meeting in a way that would make her presence, as a lawyer, of any benefit to the client.
>
> But she couldn't tell the elderly woman no, so she went to the meeting anyway. The three of them—the young lawyer who was completely out of

her depth, the government employee who was used to more routine matters, and the client who said only a word or two—sorted it out in a nondescript tiny cubicle. The result: As long as the litigation was pending, the client's Social Security checks would remain the same.

After the meeting, the client expressed gratitude that seemed out of proportion for what the lawyer had done. It turned out that the lawyer's simply showing up to this single meeting—and the continuation of the monthly checks that followed—were far more important to the client than the years-long lawsuit against the loan shark, even more important to her than whose name was on the deed to the house.

Years later, the lawyer tells this story to law students as a lesson about listening to your clients and figuring out what's important to them; it may not be what you expect. We retell it here to demonstrate the importance of allowing yourself and your settled (or prescribed) ways of doing things to be interrupted.

The firm's clients were mostly businesses, and the lawyers working there spent most of their time on complex contracts to buy, sell, and finance businesses. Their meetings with clients and others were held in fancy conference rooms in business towers where the participants wore expensive suits and made million-dollar decisions. The call to go to this client's Social Security meeting was anything but ordinary and routine for a lawyer working at this law firm. But, as John Lennon famously sang, "Life is what happens to you while you're busy making other plans."[2]

Consider other ways the lawyer might have reacted to the client's call. It would have been easy for her to conclude that the client was trying to get more free representation than had been agreed to, ensnaring the lawyer into solving more of the day-to-day bureaucratic hassles she faced. In other words, she might have seen the client as trying to take advantage, to get something from her and the law firm that she wasn't entitled to. In the previous pattern about manipulative behavior (Pattern 21), we caution against such assumptions because they close down or reduce our ability to reckon with whoever or whatever is actually facing us. *Yes*, the client was trying to get more free representation than had been agreed to, *and* the reduction in Social Security payments was clearly linked to the theft of her house.

Even without any sense of being taken advantage of, the lawyer would have been acting well within expected and typical ways of dealing with this situation had she told the client she could not represent her at the Social Security meeting. Saying no could be justified by the lawyer as adherence to the firm's habitual practices and submission to its hierarchy—and justified by the firm because its responsibility, as determined by professional rules of conduct, was limited to helping the client regain ownership of her home, the only legal matter the firm had accepted.

Similar ways of limiting the scope of services one is able or willing to provide can apply in other employment and professional settings as well. Such limits serve important purposes in setting boundaries and expectations. It is appropriate for a doctor to tell a patient that they need to see another kind of specialist for their condition. Professionals generally have lanes—a corporate lawyer is not a Social Security specialist; an orthopedist does not treat a troubling mole; a history teacher does not give math homework. And it goes without saying that a lawyer is not a doctor, a teacher is not a social worker, a doctor is not a priest. Yet occasionally someone—client, student, patient—may present a problem or ask for a sort of help that falls outside the lines of professional services.

It is not uncommon, for example, for doctors who treat persons with potentially terminal conditions to encounter a patient who seeks to draw them into a conversation about spiritual matters, because that is what's most on the patient's mind as they confront the prospect of death. Engaging in deep discussions of spiritual concerns is not within a physician's professional sphere of expertise; doctors are not trained to be spiritual counselors. On the other hand, they are expected to manifest care toward their patients and, in addition to being doctors, they are human beings in relation with other human beings. There is a significant difference, in care and humaneness, between shutting down such a conversation as soon as it arises and instead listening to the concerns, allowing the interruption of routine and expectation to happen. What then results could range from the doctor's simply holding the concerns with the patient to gently guiding the patient toward someone better prepared to counsel them, using questions like, "Who do you usually talk with about these sorts of things?" or, when it seems appropriate, "Would you like to speak with the hospital chaplain?" In any case, the doctor's allowing that rupture of self and of professional routine can help the patient, like Matt Horowitz (Pattern 3), feel heard and known—welcome in the world as it is now.

Someone will at times bring to us a problem or a question we don't expect, for which we do not feel prepared, or which seems to ask for more than we think we have to give. The temptation to push them away, as the TSA agent did, or to abruptly evade the question, as a physician may, can be strong. But, unless we allow ourselves and our routines to be interrupted by that call—let ourselves pick up the phone (recall the metaphor of the ringing telephone in Pattern 3)—we won't know if the call really is for us and that we are being asked to learn something new about our role and our capabilities. Even asked to learn that we do have a way to respond well or the particular skill needed, or the good sense to know to whom the concerns may be better directed.

In the story above, it was not just the lawyer's work routine that was interrupted. It was her view of her role and of herself in that role. She didn't know how her presence could be beneficial at the meeting with the Social Security agent, what she could bring "as a lawyer" to the meeting. There was no contract to interpret, no court document to file. She didn't even know the relevant law. But what she learned by attending the meeting—answering the client's call—was that lawyers play lots of roles: trusted adviser, companion through difficult or complex encounters, listener, explainer.

An ethics of welcome insists we allow ourselves to be interrupted by other persons in order to hear their questions, consider their needs, reevaluate our priorities and capabilities, adapt, and respond. We often regard and react to an interruption as something negative: a time-waster, a distraction, an obstacle. But we can instead learn to think of it as life happening to us: an opportunity, a new focus, a call that opens us to welcome and respond.

This is the sense in which ethicist Laurie Zoloth, using Levinas' language, writes that the other person's "interruption defines and authorizes our being."[3] It brings us into life as it happens.

The most important role for each of us is the role of human being in relation with other human beings (Pattern 3). Sometimes it takes an interruption for us to see that.

Look up. Listen up. Pick up the phone.

Notes

1 Daniel F. Chambliss, *Beyond Caring: Hospitals, Nurses, and the Social Organization of Ethics* (University of Chicago Press, Chicago, 1996).
2 Although it appears in John Lennon's 1980 song, "Beautiful Boy," this phrase did not originate with him. Its exact origins are unknown, but it is often attributed to journalist and cartoonist Allen Saunders.
3 Laurie Zoloth, "I Want You," 210.

23

Put People before Principles

The principles by which we order our moral lives can only be comprehended by welcoming others.

One of our students shared this story about her brother "Jake." The events happened a few decades ago.

> When Jake was three years old, he was hospitalized because of symptoms that were eventually confirmed to be due to cystic fibrosis. After telling Jake's parents about their son's condition, the doctors said they were going to Jake's hospital room to explain the diagnosis to him and would also tell him the average life expectancy of a child with cystic fibrosis, which at that time was about 12 years. The doctors stated that it was their duty to explain these facts to Jake.
>
> The parents balked. They worried about the trauma Jake was already experiencing in the unfamiliar setting of the hospital. It was his first hospitalization, first experience with large groups of medical professionals, and he was fearful and confused. The parents said they would explain the diagnosis to Jake in their own way, at their own time. But the doctors continued to insist that they were the ones to do this. They considered it their responsibility. They expressed concern that Jake's parents would not tell him about his shortened life expectancy, information they felt was crucial for the child to know.
>
> *At age three?*

Telling the truth is surely an important and reliable guide for moral behavior; honesty really is the best policy, usually.[1] On the other hand, truth can be a blunt and sometimes brutal weapon when wielded indiscriminately. We are all likely to have experience with wrestling over whether and how to answer honestly questions that make us squirm. Questions in our personal lives like,

"Honey, how do you think I look in this?" or "Granny, are my parents getting a divorce?" Questions in our professional lives like, "Professor, can you write me a strong recommendation for law school?" or "Doctor, what are my chances?" How do we honor our loyalty to our moral principles—in this case, to telling the truth—and, at the same time, attend well to the person asking the question?

Much has been written about distinguishing between truthfulness and factual accuracy, about whether one must tell the truth to someone who intends to use the information to harm others, and so on. Rather than review such arguments here, however, we instead want to focus on the role of welcome in helping us discern what the principle of truth-telling is asking of us in a particular situation.

Disclosing information to patients is, of course, an instance of truth-telling. In general, nurses and doctors are expected to be truthful when talking with patients, but that simple assumption leaves unasked, and unanswered, a multitude of questions, among them: Which facts should be revealed when, how, and to whom? What other, as yet unconsidered, truths may be important to the patient? What is the patient's level of understanding of the information? What harm may be done by the telling, and how can it be avoided? Note, too, that these questions are equally relevant to nonmedical instances of truth-telling—just substitute "other person" for "patient."

There are numerous healthcare practices in which such questions play an important role. Among the most complicated is the task of providing patients with a prognosis, a prediction about the likely course of their illness, often including whether it may at some point result in death. The process of providing diagnostic and related prognostic information to patients is clearly better today than it used to be. In the 1960s, for example, it was still commonplace for physicians to avoid telling patients that they had cancer for fear they would collapse in despair. No longer are test results commonly withheld from patients or families, nor serious arguments made that it would be better for patients to be kept in the dark about their conditions. Yet, there are still significant deficiencies in the ways in which some practitioners present this information to patients. To be fair, getting this right—figuring out what amount and level of information and which method of delivery is most helpful to a patient or desired by them—can be a remarkably difficult thing to do.

Prognoses are not reliably precise calculations. Plus, healthcare professionals can be hurried, forgetful, or sometimes even uninformed themselves. But what is of interest for the point being made in this pattern are the ways in which *devotion to the principle itself* can result in the truth teller's overlooking the intended recipient of this truth, such as three-year-old Jake, failing to take sufficient notice of the actual person whose well-being is at stake, *the person the principle is designed to serve.*

We can reasonably have different views on how and when, with what degree of detail, in what words, and with what forms of encouragement and comfort, information might best have been provided to Jake. We can also differ about the age at which certain information can or should be shared, and how the appropriate age may vary depending on the individual child. But we can surely agree that it was unreasonable for the doctors to insist that the disclosure happen right then, that they were the ones to decide which information to disclose and how it should be done, and, further, that they were the only ones who could deliver it. Their overstepping seems so egregious that we are led to wonder, "What were they thinking?" But, once we set aside our astonishment at their insistence on having their way and our bafflement at their apparent ignorance of a three-year-old's cognitive capacities, we can conjure a charitable interpretation: They must have sincerely believed that their proposed action was morally required as part of their responsibility to tell the truth.

Some of the routines in our lives are not simply protocols that make certain daily activities easier (see Pattern 22) but are commitments to models of thought and behavior that guide our lives more generally—often identified as our *principles*. In order to fulfill our responsibilities to other people consistently, we rely upon ideal standards—honesty, respect, integrity, environmental awareness, and others—that we have taken on as settled understandings, even rules, about how to live a moral life. We keep these tools at the ready to help us see what should be done, how we should act when we come upon a new or newly challenging situation, with all its many facets, mysteries, and entanglements. With guiding principles to call upon, we can avoid unconsidered ad hoc actions and unexamined habits of practice, and instead follow pathways devised with some careful forethought.

However, although these pathways have been identified or developed to help us carry out our responsibilities to others, we may fail to meet our obligations if we follow the guidelines inflexibly, by rote, without imagination or curiosity. That is, as persons who want to be welcoming, we cannot act as though we are responsible to the principles or ideals themselves, rather than to the people they are intended to serve, including ourselves.

In a best-selling guide for young adults, Hal Runkel cautions that we *should* be more loyal to our principles than we are to other people; his emphasis is on not letting our commitment to someone *override* our moral compass. If a friend wants us to help them steal a car/lie to escape punishment/profit from insider trading, we should put our adherence to moral rules firmly above allegiance to this friendship.[2] We have no argument with that.

Rather, in this pattern we are making a significantly different point: The moral rules that govern our direct interactions with each other can be rightly interpreted and followed only when we allow the other persons involved to guide our understanding of the rule in this particular situation. It is in that sense that actual people must take precedence over abstract principles. This does not mean that the person with whom we engage should be allowed to subvert or cause us to abandon our principles, but rather that it is what we learn by welcoming that person that enables us to discern whether and how certain principles apply and where they lead us in this moment. This, then, is another way of talking about the primacy of welcome: welcoming the other person necessarily precedes and informs our awareness of how personal moral commitments may be relevant to and perhaps at stake in an encounter.

Telling the truth cannot be a "truth dump." That term generally refers to saying too much, too fast, too soon, and includes the judgment that the teller is relieving himself or herself of a burden (think dump truck) instead of considering the recipient's experience or needs. Physician and sociologist Nicholas Christakis explains the term: "Physicians call the practice of unduly rapid or excessively comprehensive prognostication 'terminal candor' or 'truth dumping,' and they deplore it as irresponsible, though they recognize that it is not uncommon."[3] Persons of any age can experience a "truth dump" as traumatic and harmful, leading those who criticize the practice to describe it as "hitting them over the head" or "bludgeoning" them with information.

It may seem to physicians doing the dumping that they are fulfilling their duties, but they are in fact dodging them. Christakis writes,

> Truth dumping amounts to an avoidance of responsibility, in several senses: physicians thereby avoid having to engage in a lengthier, more human interaction, avoid having to face or discuss the limitations of their ability, and avoid having to address the implications of such bad news for patients. They can, however, conveniently claim that they have told the patient "the truth."[4]

The quotation marks around "the truth" in that last sentence are telling. They are a marker for the recognition that what is being dumped on the patient is the physician's conception of what constitutes truth. Doctors may be mistaken about that in a number of ways. One is that what they regard as factual at the time of telling may no longer be true even months later. Another is that the facts being told may not be the truth the patient is concerned about. In the rush to be sure a patient understands that their condition will, say, result in their death within months, the doctor may miss the opportunity to provide particular truths that the patient really wants to know: We can control your pain; you will most likely make it to your grandson's wedding; we will be at your side till the end. Ensuring that the person takes precedence over the principle of truth-telling allows the welcomer—the truth teller—to discern more accurately which important truths need to be told, to sense more clearly how to say what needs saying, and to come closer to meeting their own ideal of honesty.

An epilogue to Jake's story: fortunately, the doctors did not prevail. Instead, his parents virtually kicked the doctors out of their son's hospital room, preventing the intended truth dump. Jake did, in time, learn of his diagnosis and also the presumed prognosis which, because of continuing advances in treatment, has become markedly better over time. (As of this writing, the average life expectancy for persons with cystic fibrosis is forty-five to fifty years.) When we learned of his story, Jake was in his late twenties, managing his disease well and living a rich and busy life.

Another common moral principle, closely related to the commitment to tell the truth, is that of showing *respect* for others. We speak of respect often in this book; failures of welcome are usually also failures of respect. When we show respect, just as when we offer welcome, we are regarding and honoring someone *as they are right now* (Pattern 11). As with truth-telling, the problem lies not with the principle of respect itself but with an inflexible interpretation and adherence that does not attend sufficiently to the reality of the person to whom we wish to show respect.

Respect for an adult generally includes, for example, allowing them to make their own decisions about their medical care, whereas respect for a two-year-old child would include *not* allowing them to choose whether to take their prescribed medicine. But even such a simple distinction as this one becomes complicated when the adult no longer has the expected reasoning capacities of a mature human being. What does it mean to respect an adult who has trouble thinking, trouble ordering their life and their behaviors?

Consider persons with "trouble thinking" due to advanced Alzheimer's Disease or some other form of severe dementia. In general, respecting an adult entails honoring their status (or dignity) as a mature human being who is not to be lied to—truth-telling being a central manifestation of respect—nor treated like a child. Yet, persons who live with and care for adults with dementia attest to the distress that can result from letting that definition of respect govern interactions. For example, a widower who keeps asking for his wife can be forced to reexperience daily the grief of her death by well-meaning attendants who insist upon respecting his dignity by telling him that his wife is dead each time he asks.

Rebecca Mead, in the *New Yorker*, and Pam Belluck, in the *New York Times*, have reported on evolving concepts about caring for individuals with advanced Alzheimer's Disease, ideas that set aside rigid rules, including some abstract understandings of respect, and focus instead on helping residents feel better and more content. According to Mead's account, this innovative approach was embraced by a retirement community in Arizona where some traditional procedures (such as physical and chemical restraints) were abandoned and some unusual practices (including some that at first glance may seem "disrespectful") were adopted. She writes,

> Although it once was standard practice in nursing homes to "re-orient" residents who became confused about the identities of staff members, [the director of education and research at the Arizona facility] said that it is more comforting to residents if staff members play along with their delusions. One former resident, a retired dentist, was often distracted from incipient distress by a female staff member requesting a dental exam; she then opened her mouth, so that he could peer inside.[5]

Another resident was given a doll to care for. At first, even the director cited above objected to this intervention as disrespectful, considering "the doll an 'undignified' and demeaning security blanket." But she changed her mind when she saw the pleasure the resident got from caring for it and how calm she became when she had the doll with her. She would even eat a few bites of food on her own once she first fed the doll.[6]

The resident's care for the doll may have been a manifestation of her deep commitment to being a mother or of a treasured experience of caregiving, the details of which she can no longer recall. Whatever its meaning to her, it seems clear that allowing her to experience and express care and devotion honored an essential part of who she had been and still was. When the staff provided the resident with the doll, it was not because they believed her dignity no longer mattered or that she no longer merited respect. Quite the contrary. By their actions, they were showing the utmost respect for her by enabling her to express her own deeply held values, still intact and meaningful despite the ravages of her dementia, and thereby to assert her dignity.

To be clear, ethical principles like truth-telling and respect serve a crucial, indispensable role in our moral lives. But they, like all abstract notions, require examination and interpretation if they are to be relevant and effective in the concrete situations that call us to be ethical people. The person to whom we want to tell the truth, the person to whom we intend to show respect, is our essential guide to comprehending how we can fulfill the principles to which we are devoted.

Staff members at the Arizona retirement community can carry out their responsibility to care for their residents because they welcome them as they are. They can see that telling the truth to the widower does not require them to remind him, multiple times each day, of the fact that his wife is dead. Rather, they can offer, and reoffer, the simple truth that she's not here right now, assuaging his momentary anxiety. They can see that respecting the distraught dentist or bereft grandmother does not mean constantly reminding them of their thinking problems, but instead recognizing the deeper core of their identities. Offering a mouth to examine or a doll to care for can be the highest form of respect because it is a reassurance that they are still welcome, as they are, in the world as it is now.

Be loyal to your principles, in all their complexity and strength, by being open to learning from those whom you welcome what the rules mean in this moment and require in response.

Notes

1. It should be noted that "do not lie" ("do not say that which you know is not true") is generally held to be a near-absolute dictum, not a prima facie rule. Telling the truth, however, is not a simple corollary of "do not lie." It is a more complex undertaking that does not lend itself easily to being an inflexible command. See, for example, Sissela Bok, *Lying: Moral Choice in Public and Private Life*, 2nd ed. (Vintage, New York, 1999).
2. Hal Runkel, *Choose Your Own Adulthood: A Small Book about the Small Choices That Make the Biggest Difference* (Greenleaf Book Group Press, Austin, 2016), 37–43.
3. Nicholas A. Christakis, *Death Foretold: Prophecy and Prognosis in Medical Care* (University of Chicago Press, Chicago,1999), 109.
4. Christakis, *Death Foretold*, 109.

5   Rebecca Mead, "The Sense of an Ending," *The New Yorker*, May 13, 2013, 92–103, https://www.newyorker.com/magazine/2013/05/20/the-sense-of-an-ending-2
6   Pam Belluck, "Giving Alzheimer's Patients Their Way, Even Chocolate," *The New York Times*, December 31, 2010, https://www.nytimes.com/2011/01/01/health/01care.html

24

Help Others Welcome You

We may, at times, encounter persons who appear not to welcome us in return. Although this can be a clear signal that no meaningful connection is possible—and should be respected as such—it may also be the case that, by our own welcoming approaches, we can help the other person welcome us.

Welcome is a mutual obligation (see Pattern 7), but the particular person we seek to welcome may not appear to be welcoming toward us. This can happen for any number of reasons. For one, it may be due to circumstances, not something about us. Perhaps the person we want to welcome is preoccupied with some trouble in their life or fearful about the situation at hand, like someone awaiting a crucial job interview. When this is the case, recognizing that the perceived rejection of our welcome is not personal can allow us to continue our welcoming practices (like calling the person by their name, paying attention to them, listening to what they have to say, and the like) while not pressing for or expecting any matching response.

These practices may help the other person move into a more open and responsive posture but, whether or not this happens, our primary task is simply to *be* welcoming. This takes work, to be sure, because in the face of what can feel like rejection, it's easy for us to be reactive rather than responsive—to snap back, as it were—or to judge the person before us as just one of a type. As always, it takes practice to be consistently welcoming.

And sometimes it *is* personal. The unwelcoming stance of the other person may indeed be a direct reaction to us, to our self-presentation, to what we appear to represent. It may have roots in prejudice, anger, condescension, past experience, or fear. In such a situation, it can be very challenging to sustain welcoming behaviors. We can try, for instance, to invite the other into our world (Pattern 6), but once that invitation has been roundly rejected, it is natural to think we're done. We tried. We did our part. They didn't meet us halfway.

An ethics of welcome, however, is not about meeting people halfway. It is not transactional, not based on quid pro quo contractual norms, where "this" is given in exchange for "that." Welcome doesn't measure or compare how far we each came. We don't meet each other in the middle, which would mean that each of us steps out of our own world but not into the other's. Instead, as we discussed in Pattern 7 using the image of Venn diagrams, what is sought is an intersection of worlds. For that, it doesn't matter who has to travel how far. This is yet another way in which welcome stretches us.

So, if we don't get to give up on the possibility of a welcoming connection just because the other person appears unwilling to join us, then what are we to do? Because welcome is not coercive, we must accept the other person's refusal of our welcome (Pattern 7). But we also have to determine if what we think sounds like a no is, in fact, a no. That is, we have to strike a careful, attentive balance among our obligations to be welcoming, to respect others as they are—including their refusals and animosities—and to respect, protect, and welcome ourselves. The following story, which happened around 2012, allows us to explore what such a balancing might look like.

First, a disclaimer: This story was reported to one of us by a small group of medical students who were present for the interaction. We know only what they related, what they saw and heard filtered through their interpretation of the events. Had we been there, we might have understood things differently, but since we were not, what we have to say about the two "players" in this scenario—whom we call Ms. Smythe and Dr. Wilson—can be applicable only to the quasi-fictional characters in the story as related, not to the actual persons involved.

> Jean Smythe, an elderly White woman and nursing home resident, had for several years been cared for by the physician who was the nursing home's medical director and the nurse practitioner who worked with that doctor, both also White women. Ms. Smythe was especially close to and trusted the nurse practitioner, whom she saw much more frequently than the doctor. That doctor has now retired, and the new medical director is Jacqueline Wilson, a geriatric specialist. Dr. Wilson, accompanied by three or four

medical students, came to visit Ms. Smythe for the first time. As the doctor introduced herself, Ms. Smythe said, "You're Black!" Dr. Wilson replied, "Yes, I'm Black as Black can be," and then asked about the pain the patient was experiencing.

During the rest of the visit, Ms. Smythe made no further comments but, as Dr. Wilson was finishing up by writing a prescription for pain medication, she asked whether she could choose her own doctor at the nursing home. Dr. Wilson explained that she could, but that she was the only doctor who worked with the nurse practitioner Ms. Smythe liked so much. Ms. Smythe could have a doctor from outside the facility—Dr. Wilson said she would be happy to refer her to one—but she might not be seen as frequently and would no longer be able to receive her care from the nurse practitioner. If that's what she wanted, Dr. Wilson said, she would make the referral that afternoon. Ms. Smythe said that was what she wanted, and so the referral was made as soon as Dr. Wilson left the patient's room.

When they later recounted this experience, the medical students reported their shock and dismay that such blatant prejudice still existed. They expressed admiration for Dr. Wilson for treating Ms. Smythe calmly and with respect despite her attitude toward the doctor. Indeed, they admired Dr. Wilson for treating her at all. At least one of them questioned whether they would have been tempted, had they been in Dr. Wilson's shoes, to ignore the patient's report of pain and fail to prescribe for it. That is, the students' reactions were so powerful that some of them seemed willing, at least in theory, either to abandon the patient mid-appointment or to intentionally provide her with poor care, both clear violations of basic professional norms. (We return to the medical students' response to this episode in Pattern 27.)

Their perspective seemed to be that of justice: Ms. Smythe had treated Dr. Wilson unfairly and unequally on account of race, and Dr. Wilson would therefore have been justified had she walked out of the room and refused to treat her at all. If we understand justice to be "what is deserved," then that is what they believed Ms. Smythe deserved. Anything Dr. Wilson did above and beyond that was to be praised as gracious, generous, and charitable.

In our focus on welcome, however, we wish to examine the story in more depth. Justice is an exceedingly narrow lens through which to view human interactions—and perhaps particularly medical care encounters, in which "what is deserved" is rarely what patients seek or receive or what practitioners strive to provide. It is difficult to know what justice might even look like when patients can find themselves so abjectly dependent on others. "Can I choose my own doctor?" Ms. Smythe asks because she actually does not know and may suspect she won't be allowed to.

Before going further, it is important to emphasize that there is far too little information available, too much unknown about Dr. Wilson and Ms. Smythe—their life experiences, expectations, and, in the case of Ms. Smythe, her cognitive capacities—to draw any moral judgments about this situation. The issue here is not determining where right and wrong lie. It is, rather, seeing what may become possible when we practice being welcoming and allowing ourselves to be interrupted and changed, even just a bit, by our encounters.

Certainly, the obligations of welcome would seem to call on Ms. Smythe to do better at welcoming Dr. Wilson. But the story, as related, suggests that, whether she intended to be welcoming or not, she was stopped short, first by her startled reaction to Dr. Wilson's being Black, and then by the doctor's quick shift to medical questions. By the students' report, Ms. Smythe did not say anything negative about Black people or Black doctors, nor did she seem reluctant to interact with Dr. Wilson. One can *infer* prejudice from both her initial comment and her later request to change doctors, but we don't actually know if she made prejudgments about Dr. Wilson, as a person or as a physician, on the basis of her skin color or whether, if she did, those judgments were open to change. We don't know if her decision to choose a different doctor was due to deep-seated racial prejudice or to Dr. Wilson's brusque reaction to her thoughtless comment.

Welcome is a manifestation of the desire, the intention to be in the presence of another person and, when possible, to forge a connection, no matter how limited in depth or duration, within which each person can be heard and known to some extent. In order to fulfill the obligation to welcome, sometimes we have to help others to welcome us, and that may mean getting past initial reactions—ours and theirs—to look for possible points of contact. Plus, the respect that is integral to welcome insists that we have positive expectations of each other. Showing that kind of respect may require us to linger a moment longer, after a first negative reaction, in the hope (and expectation) of a more welcoming approach from ourselves and from the person we want to welcome. Respect asks Ms. Smythe to stop and consider Dr. Wilson again—and it asks Dr. Wilson to stop and consider Ms. Smythe again.

We don't know if Dr. Wilson interpreted Ms. Smythe's blurting, "You're Black!" as a rejection of the possibility of connection or of the doctor personally. We were told only that she moved on. But what if it wasn't a rejection at all? What might have been the outcome if Dr. Wilson had stepped beyond her understandable reaction to Ms. Smythe's remark and had, however cautiously, explored Ms. Smythe's astonishment with her? Perhaps Dr. Wilson could have simply responded, "Yes, I am," and then waited expectantly, hopefully, to see what Ms. Smythe might say next—or have gone a bit further to invite a conversation: "You seem surprised. Is this something we can talk about?"

Ms. Smythe, given the opportunity, may have responded with her own tentative attempt at welcome: "This is all so new to me. I've never known a Black doctor. It's going to take me a while to get used to you, but I'll try." Considering Ms. Smythe's age and situation, we can even wonder whether she might have said something like, "Please forgive me. I've just never had this experience before, and anymore I just seem to blurt out whatever I'm thinking. I'm delighted to meet you." That is, Dr. Wilson's choice to continue being welcoming may have opened up meaningful possibilities for rapport.

Of course, an inviting, welcoming response by Dr. Wilson to Ms. Smythe's initial remark also carries a real risk of even more discomfort, the sort of serious unpleasantness that the doctor appears to have been trying to avoid. Ms. Smythe could have revealed a determined animosity, rejecting Dr. Wilson's overtures with insults and viciousness. In that case, the doctor would be justified in ceasing her attempts to establish a relationship and in ending the encounter as quickly as possible after fulfilling her basic professional obligations.

Whether Dr. Wilson should take such a risk is for her to decide, not us. There can indeed be costs to welcome, and *only* the welcomer—in this case, Dr. Wilson—can assess them and then choose to pay or not. It is neither for us to decide nor for us to judge the decision-maker. We consider further this matter of assessing the risks and bearing the costs of welcome in Pattern 25, where we continue to examine the interaction between Dr. Wilson and Ms. Smythe, in parallel with a story in which the hostility of the one being welcomed is unmistakable.

For now, we emphasize what may be gained by including among our welcoming practices ways of helping the other person welcome us. Let's not forget what Ms. Smythe lost in her encounter with Dr. Wilson. She lost the ability to have more frequent doctor's visits by selecting a physician who was not the institution's medical director, and she lost the care of the nurse practitioner with whom she had built a close relationship over the years. For an elderly person in a nursing facility, such losses are significant and consequential, not to be taken lightly. Moreover, she missed out on the possibility of expanding her world, broadening her outlook a bit by forming a connection with Dr. Wilson. Had Dr. Wilson reached out in welcome just a bit more, it is possible that things could have turned out much better for Ms. Smythe—and also, perhaps, for the doctor, who stood at least some chance of learning that she was *not*, in fact, being rejected because of her race and who would likely have earned even more respect from her students as they learned from her valuable lessons about responsive, caring attention.

In situations when the refusal of a welcome is not clear, if possible, take a moment of expectant silence or gentle exploration to see if you can help the other person welcome you.

Part IV

How Far Do We Have to Go?

Throughout this book, we discuss what being welcoming asks of us, including that we be open to others and responsive rather than reactive; that we allow ourselves to be moved by others and then move toward them in some fashion; that we break out of old modes of stereotyping others and imagining our own stories about their lives and motives; and that we attentively practice being welcoming. In Part IV, we consider what welcome "asks of us" in another sense of that phrase: What do we risk when we open ourselves to someone else? What might it cost us to be welcoming? What limits, if any, can we set on this obligation?

25

Welcome Can Be Costly

The potential costs of welcoming another person can sometimes be too high for us to engage in welcoming actions. More often, we can responsibly balance our obligation to welcome and our obligation to care well for ourselves.

The risks entailed in being welcoming are the unpredictable chances we take when we allow ourselves to be open and stay open to another person. How such openness may affect us and what it may require of us—some real discomfort, for example, or disruption of our opinions, attitudes, habits—are potential costs of being welcoming.

Some of the costs entailed by being welcoming may seem relatively trivial. The Ritchies, the "Australian Angels" introduced in the first pattern, gave up some relaxed afternoons and a lot of tea. But, in fact, apparently minor expenditures related to time, energy, and inconvenience can add up and are not to be taken lightly. The effort it takes to be "on" all the time—especially on occasions when our intention and attention lag behind our sense of obligation, when we don't feel like being open to this person or, maybe, to anybody right now—can be exhausting, particularly when some of the practices are new to us.

Of course, the costs to the Ritchies were surely greater than those inconveniences. Reaching out to persons contemplating suicide had to have taken a significant emotional toll on them. There must have been times when Don and Moya whispered, "Not again," as they saw someone approaching the cliff's edge and realized they were heading out toward another difficult conversation with a troubled soul, wrenching in its evocation of despair and grief. Being open to others can expose us to their emotional turmoil and cause our own.

Underlying all the aspects of welcome we explore is the recognition that being welcoming has an impact on us, that each encounter changes us in some way (a topic discussed in Pattern 14)—and change is rarely cost-free. Being truly open to someone cannot help but alter the way we perceive their life and perhaps our perception of life in general, as well as our perception of ourselves. We learn something in every encounter, each time we enter the room, each time we stay. There is a lot of positive personal growth that can happen as we do this, as we open ourselves to the endlessly abundant ways of being human. Sometimes that personal growth feels good as it is happening. But sometimes it doesn't. The realignments such growth may call for in us—for example, when we have to shift away from old habits of reaction—can be accompanied by feelings of confusion and shame, and may spur defensiveness and resistance. Some fundamental alterations of perspective can feel like betrayals of old loyalties. It's not easy, not painless.

There are also the costs of having our welcome be rejected. Think of the grief and helplessness the Ritchies are likely to have experienced when someone turned away from their open hands and jumped from that cliff anyway. Even refusals less dramatic and terrible than those can exact a toll, particularly when the rebuff seems not simply indifferent but deliberate and personal (see Pattern 24).

In this pattern, we delve more deeply into the potential costliness of welcome in order to tackle hard questions: What are we to do when welcoming someone risks not just rejection, but hurt, humiliation, vitriol from the other person? Addressing these sorts of risks leads us, in Pattern 26, to consider situations in which the cost of welcoming a particular person seems so extraordinarily high that it is too much to expect.

It is important to be clear about one crucial aspect of taking risks as we welcome others: *If reaching out in welcome to someone appears to entail a real possibility of physical violence, to oneself or others, then it must not be attempted.* Common sense, as well as the obligation to care for ourselves and others who may be in danger, require us to step away and take protective measures, not to step forward in welcome. In all that follows, we are describing situations in which there is no discernible threat of such violence.

We focus in this pattern on the risks of being rejected or even directly attacked because of some aspect of our personal identity such as our skin color, ethnicity, religion, gender performance, or the like. But, before we take up that discussion, we first consider briefly a risk that does not have to do with intentional negativity from the one we welcome, but arises simply from the experience of opening ourselves to the truth of someone else's life.

As we assert many times in this book, welcome requires paying attention, which includes listening carefully to others' stories, inviting revelations that allow us to know one another as the unique persons we are and that, in the case of professional encounters, enable understanding that is crucial for the work of therapists, lawyers, social workers, clergypersons, physicians, and the like. But the raw details of some persons' lives can be distressing in the extreme. They may evoke feelings of sadness, outrage, or disgust, or bring to mind similar events in our own past.

As we listen to others' stories, we are always at risk of hearing our own stories coming back at us, some with the power to re-inflict old trauma or current pain. For example, caregivers of various sorts, at least as often as those to whom they give care, are also children of alcoholic parents, survivors of sexual abuse, active or recovering addicts, trapped in loveless marriages, and so on. We may also hear tales utterly foreign to our experience and frightful in the previously unimagined possibilities of hurt and harm they reveal. Fear of what one might hear and be called upon to experience vicariously may keep some would-be welcomers from being as open as they might wish to be, from asking the next question that could open a door they really don't want to step through.

In most cases, the costs that come with hearing others' stories, daunting though they may be, are part of what we accept when we set out to be welcoming people generally, and especially if we elect to take on the privileged position of a caregiving practitioner. It is incumbent upon the teachers and advisers of future clergy, therapists, healthcare providers—of anyone entering a vocation that adds particular professional obligations of open responsiveness to the universal personal obligation of welcome—to make that fact plain, discuss the real and imagined perils of exposing oneself to such human realities, and help their students learn how to protect themselves without closing down.

These are lessons valuable for all of us, professional listeners and all others, as we seek to be more reliably welcoming persons. It may be that, for some of us, protecting ourselves calls for therapeutic interventions that enable us to come to grips with episodes in our own lives that continue to have the power to disrupt our interactions with others. But for most of us, most of the time, being able to remain open while shielding ourselves from the effects of the stories we hear means learning to recognize the existential boundaries between ourselves and those we attend to. We can remind ourselves that the story we are hearing is not our own and that the other's suffering, however closely embraced, does not become our own suffering, at least not in the same way or with the same intensity. This boundary recognition is also essential for keeping our perspective clear. Imagining that someone else's situation is *actually* happening to us when we hear about it can trigger any number of unhelpful, even irresponsible reactions in us. For example, the judges who heard the case of Elizabeth Bouvia (presented in Pattern 12) appear to have been so disturbed by picturing themselves in Bouvia's position, "lying helplessly in bed, unable to care for herself," that they could not focus on Bouvia herself nor bring themselves to consider the possibility that her continued existence could be valuable to her and to others.

Becoming capable of staying present for the most harrowing stories is one thing. It is quite another to think of continuing to welcome someone who is expressing reprehensible biases against us or against people and things that matter to us. Physician-poet Dannie Abse, in his poem "Case History,"[1] writes about just such a situation, in which it is strikingly clear that the obligation to welcome others (specifically, in this case, a healthcare practitioner's obligation to welcome his patient) may at times carry a high cost.

"Most Welshmen are worthless,
an inferior breed, doctor."
He did not know I was Welsh.
Then he praised the architects
of the German death-camps--
did not know I was a Jew.
He called liberals, "White blacks",
and continued to invent curses.

When I palpated his liver
I felt the soft liver of Goering;
when I lifted my stethoscope
I heard the heartbeats of Himmler;
when I read his encephalograph
I thought, "Sieg heil, mein Fuhrer."

In the clinic's dispensary
red berry of black bryony,
cowbane, deadly nightshade, deathcap.
Yet I prescribed for him
as if he were my brother.

Later that night I must have slept
on my arm: momentarily
my right hand lost its cunning.

In that final line of the poem, Abse is echoing the words of Psalm 137—"If I forget thee, O Jerusalem, let my right hand forget her cunning"—in which the Jewish psalm-singer, in exile from Israel, offers up the skill of his hand on the harp (his vocation and the way he makes his living) as a fitting consequence should he falter in his loyalty to his faith and his people. Abse evokes this image to articulate the price the doctor felt he paid for betraying allegiances so deeply held as to be inseparable from self. Is this what welcome asks of us?

No. Betrayal of self is not one of the requirements of welcome; in fact, it is a violation of the obligation to welcome ourselves. However, a welcoming orientation does ask that we cultivate a clear-eyed awareness of what is at stake and be willing to take some risks.

In Pattern 24, we offer a story about Dr. Wilson, a Black physician encountering an elderly White patient, Ms. Smythe, who seems startled by her Black skin and eventually asks to be referred to another doctor. It is instructive to compare the ways in which Abse's fictional physician (who may or may not be a stand-in for Dr. Abse himself) and Dr. Wilson responded to their patients and the price each paid or refused to pay, and then to consider what an ethics of welcome would propose instead.

The physician in the poem notes the prejudicial remarks and also sees that the patient is ignorant of the doctor's ethnic origin, faith tradition, and political inclinations which, unlike Dr. Wilson's Blackness, are not outwardly apparent. He does not respond to the remarks aloud; he does not inform the patient that he is Welsh and Jewish, nor does he challenge his bigotry. Although his angry internal response is clear—he envisions the patient as an avatar of Nazism and contemplates poisoning him—his outward behavior remains professional, even fraternal. Only in the relaxation of sleep does he experience the cost: In remaining true to his perceived professional obligations, he feels he has betrayed his identifying commitments, particularly his Jewishness, and thereby has betrayed himself.

Dr. Wilson's situation is different: She is undeniably Black; her patient confronts her directly with a blunt statement of that fact—"You're Black!"—as though it were a surprise. Dr. Wilson, according to the students' account, acknowledges the truth of the observation but goes no further. When Ms. Smythe later ventures a question about switching doctors, Dr. Wilson, like Abse's physician, remains outwardly professional and efficient. Unlike the doctor in the poem, she does not tell us what this encounter felt like. She may reasonably have felt an upsurge of anger, the memory of similar past encounters, and an immediate defensive reaction against the threat of being put in a position of assumed inadequacy based solely on her skin color. This inner turmoil, likely made worse by the presence of observing medical students, may have been disturbingly familiar, the recurring consequence of being a member of a racial minority in a prejudiced society. She may have promised herself that, although she could not avoid the burden of being frequently seen as "other" and even as "inferior other," she could refuse to invite further distress by entering into a conversation about race with someone she could not trust.

By not responding directly to his patient's explicit and repellent prejudices, Abse's physician sought to uphold some of his vocational obligations, but at the cost of betraying himself. Dr. Wilson, by not responding directly to what was not yet but could have proven to be a similarly vicious level of bigotry, sought to be true to herself, but at the possible cost of betraying some of her vocational obligations. Each of them refused in some way to pay the price that they had good reason to think would be asked of them if they were to respond directly to their patient's challenges. But, in doing so, each of them incurred other costs which may have asked as much, or more, of them in the end. If we are not paying the costs of being welcoming, we are paying the costs of not being welcoming.

What if neither of them, upon reflection, is satisfied with the way the encounter turned out? How might they have responded differently? Is there a viable alternative that would allow them to honor both self and vocation without incurring unbearable costs? We think there is. In Pattern 18, where we explore issues of self-presentation, we discuss certain obligations that being welcoming imposes, including the responsibility *to be prepared* for the possibility of disturbing interactions that challenge one's personal attributes and allegiances and to be ready *to deal well with them*. Here we assert that dealing well with them is generally not most fruitfully accomplished by refusal to engage, that there are potential benefits to taking the risk entailed in responding directly—while, at the same time, acknowledging that each person must reach his or her own conclusions in each situation about how much risk is acceptable.

The practice of welcoming all others entails, in principle, not only being open to hearing what may be their noxious opinions but also being prepared to respond with questions and comments that invite them to be more welcoming in their turn. What might have happened if the doctor in Abse's poem had responded to his patient's prejudices with self-disclosure and a challenging question: "I am both Welsh and Jewish. I strongly disagree with and abhor what you say. Is it possible for us to come to some understanding that would allow me to continue as your physician?" Maybe the patient would have stormed out of the office and taken himself to another doctor. Or he may have unleashed even more venom directly toward the doctor, who would then be correct to end the encounter immediately ("It is clear that we cannot work together. Do you wish me to give you names of other physicians in the area? Now please leave."). If the situation were such that the patient was in need of immediate help and there was no other source of care available, the physician's initial reply would allow him to continue by setting the terms of their continued engagement: "I'll treat you to the best of my ability, but I must insist that you stop saying such things." On the other hand, it is also possible that the doctor's directness could deflate the patient's bluster and result in, if not an apology, at least the negotiation of a truce that would allow the visit to proceed. In any case, the doctor could have remained true both to himself and to his professional obligations.

And, as we speculated in Pattern 24, what if Dr. Wilson—in response, instead of reaction, to her patient's blurting "You're Black!"—had said, "Yes, I am," and then waited expectantly and openly for what might come, or even invited a conversation with a reflective question like "Is this something we need to talk about?" Ms. Smythe may indeed have revealed a settled animosity, saying something like, "Well, I never. This will not work. Do I get to choose my doctor here?" Or she may have said something even more vicious and rejecting, leading Dr. Wilson to rightly end the encounter immediately. On the other hand, she may have apologized or in some way expressed at least some openness to this new experience.

Welcoming persons take risks. The potential costs are not negligible, and in no way do we claim that the doctors in our examples, or anyone similarly situated, should or must continue to seek a connection with someone once it has become clear just how steep the price will be. Welcoming others is an activity that is always undertaken in conjunction with *welcoming ourselves*, being attentive to our reactions, our boundaries, our limits (see Patterns 8 and 27). An ethics of welcome does not teach that the other person's needs and desires, much less their opinions and stances, must take precedence over our own in each encounter.

Thus, our purpose is not to judge those who are not willing, for perhaps very good reasons, to continue to engage with certain persons. Rather, we seek to explore possibilities of honoring, under conditions of significant conflict, both our commitments to ourselves and our loyalties—including, in some cases, our professional obligations—and our desire and intention to be welcoming. We believe that the potential benefits of this kind of risk-taking, of continuing to be open and responsive to the apparently unwelcoming, include not only a relationship formed in honesty and acceptance but also an opportunity for growth for each person in the encounter as they are compelled to look beyond stereotypes, ingrained prejudices, and reactive defenses to see the human being in front of them.

The work of interacting with and caring for and about others is an enterprise full of enduring uncertainties, shot through with awareness that the stakes may be high and the risks may be many. But, the goodness and satisfaction of that work is generally understood to be well worth its potential and actual costs. So it is with welcome, also a risky venture, also worth it.

Be prepared for the risks involved in opening yourself to someone else. Only you can decide whether the risk is too much, whether the potential cost is more than you can bear.

Note

1 Dannie Abse, *New and Collected Poems* (Hutchinson, London, 2003).

26

Managing Aversions

No One Is Unworthy of Being Welcomed

Every person can be welcomed.

In Arthur Miller's play *Death of a Salesman*, Linda Loman, the wife of the salesman whose desperate life is careening to its close, says this about him: "He's not the finest character that ever lived. But he's a human being, and a terrible thing is happening to him. So attention must be paid.... Attention, attention must be finally paid to such a person."[1]

No one is unworthy of being welcomed, of having attention paid to them.

A medical ethicist has been called to the hospital in the middle of the night to consider whether an urgently ill man, serving a life sentence for having killed his girlfriend and her young daughter, should be approved as a candidate for a new heart:[2]

> The ethicist first speaks with the patient (whose name is Rob Dwyer) in his hospital room. He reminds himself that he is obliged "to make an unbiased assessment" but writes that he is repelled and finds the experience "creepy." He has trouble disciplining his biased imaginings, as he repeatedly pictures Dwyer as a rattlesnake and composes in his mind a vivid story of Dwyer committing murder "out of rage and to satisfy an inflated sense of himself."
>
> After he leaves the patient, the ethicist meets with the medical team and argues successfully that Dwyer should be listed as a candidate for transplant, regardless of what he has done: "He's still a person . . . a person in medical need." He goes on to explain that "Our society is committed to the principle that everybody has an inherent and equal worth," and thus Dwyer deserves "equal consideration" for listing.[3]

As he leaves that meeting, a member of the team who had vehemently opposed offering Dwyer a new heart prods him to say how he feels "deep down." The ethicist replies:

"You want to know how I feel about Dwyer?... I don't care if Dwyer dies," I said. "Even a slow and painful death is okay with me. And while he's dying, maybe he could watch a video loop of [his girlfriend] and her little girl, so he could never forget that he killed them.... I'm telling you how I *feel*.... At the meeting I said what I thought was *right*."

Impediments to welcome—the things that make us reluctant to engage with someone—can be thought of as *aversions*, by which we mean some combination of past experience, present assumption, fear, and distaste that causes us to turn away rather than step forward. Each of us likely resists welcoming persons who exhibit certain characteristics. Many of us have trouble warming up to neighbors who fly offensive banners in their front yards. Most of us move away from, not toward, angry people who get in our faces with smug and obnoxious certainties. Doctors tend not to take to patients who neglect or undermine their health or won't follow recommendations. Clergy often have a hard time being available for congregants whose avid need for attention and counsel threatens to consume large amounts of time and energy. The list is long.

Elsewhere we have made clear that welcome is not synonymous with love or empathy or generosity or hospitality, though each of these concepts is related to welcome. Welcome is also not *tolerance*. Tolerance—patient endurance of an objectionable difference[4]—might at first seem to be the right way to respond when we have an aversion to someone or some group of people. But the only goal of tolerance is peace, an absence of conflict. Its goal is not connection, not understanding, not the possibility of relationship. We can be entirely tolerant of certain other persons, and thereby live in a peaceful society, but at the cost of walling ourselves off from each other, demarcating our own separate spaces, literal or figurative, in which to be and to live.

Welcome, however, is about not building walls around ourselves or others. It is the desire for the other person's presence in our lives, in our society, right now; it is about making room together, creating space to share. It requires that we examine the deeply ingrained assumptions that have generated our objections, our aversions to the person before us, and that we hold back our reactions, those spontaneous feelings that arise when we're confronted by troubling differences, feelings of fear or annoyance or anxiety or inadequacy. In holding back, we allow both ourselves and the other person to open up to the possibility of connection and, thus, to the possibility of change, even the resolution of our differences.

Of course, one of the challenges of becoming a welcoming person is that, in order to do so, we have to *want* to get beyond our aversions so that we can see and come to know the unique person whose behaviors or attributes are triggering our reaction. Fortunately, attentive practice of all those things we wish to do well (paying attention, examining our boundaries, breaking through stereotypes, and the like) has the power to diminish, over time, our antipathies. Our distaste, fear, and impatience fade, losing their ability to derail our good intentions, our good will.

Most of our aversions can be overcome in this way, but not all of them. Included in this catchall category of "aversion" are at least two sorts of impediments to welcome. One is the kind that we can get beyond if we want to—and that we have to get beyond if we want to be welcoming people. This sort responds quite well to attentive practice. We can call these aversions *remediable*. The other sort of aversions is not so easily managed. They are the ones we may not be able to get beyond, for one reason or another, not without significant danger to our mental and emotional well-being. These we can call *protective*.

Elsewhere, we present instances of what we can now recognize as *remediable aversions*, such as those mentioned above (the needy congregant, the banner-flying neighbor) and the instinctive resistance to someone who seems manipulative (discussed in Pattern 21). The recommendations we offer for getting around and beyond the stereotypes we impose on others—strategies for seeing them as they are: whole, complex persons deserving of reconsideration beyond a glancing first impression—are fully applicable to the task of remediating our aversions, which are, after all, usually a matter of categorizing someone as a member of a type we find difficult, frightening, repellent, outrageous (see Patterns 13 and 15).

Protective aversions call for a different response. These aversions tend to arise from the ravages of personal experience, and the potential costs of getting around them may be not just painful but even self-destructive. For example, someone who suffered severe physical abuse during childhood may need to strictly avoid interacting with the abuser, and perhaps also with anyone who perpetrated similar harm, in order not to have to reexperience their pain, terror, and helplessness. Hence the protective nature of resistance to being in proximity to someone who represents past or present trauma. Such aversions serve an important purpose and may justify setting limits on the welcoming actions we are willing to engage in (see Pattern 27 for further discussion of choosing to set limits on welcome). Every human being is worthy of welcome, but this does not mean that everyone can, or must, personally welcome every person.

Aversions Based on "Principle"

On the other hand, sometimes we may think that a particular aversion is protective (and, therefore, not in need of remediation), when it does not, in fact, serve that purpose. That is, sometimes our unwillingness to engage with another person is based not on our own specific experiences but on our more general indignation about what *others* have suffered because of this person (or someone similar). Outrage, not a self-protective instinct, grounds our conviction that this is someone whom we cannot personally welcome and, more, leads us to believe, wrongly, that this is someone unworthy of being welcomed by anyone. These seemingly "principled" aversions are, in fact, remediable.

In the story presented above, the ethicist-narrator clearly describes an aversion to Dwyer, and it appears to be of this sort. The story does not reveal anything of the ethicist's own past to explain how his encounter with Dwyer would be unusually painful or traumatic—anything that would qualify his aversion as "protective." Instead, it is presented as objectively reasonable, something Dwyer deserves. And, indeed, Dwyer has engaged in reprehensible acts. Feeling an aversion to him, even a strong or almost overwhelming aversion, is something we can all probably understand.

On some accounts of ethics, the ethicist's willingness nonetheless to list Dwyer as a heart transplant candidate can be seen as admirable. And in some ways, it is. Though he detests Dwyer, his commitment to the principle of equal regard—to considering every person to be of equal value to every other person—is so unwavering that he follows it *regardless of his feelings*.

But an ethics of welcome requires a different way of thinking about the ethicist's conflict between his feelings and his principles, between his feelings and his actions. When we find ourselves in situations like this, we have to reconsider our principles—Are we really committed to the formulations we profess? Have we understood them sufficiently? Are we applying them with care?—or do the hard work of challenging our feelings, or perhaps both (see Patterns 3 and 14 for discussions of integrity).

Here, the ethicist professes his commitment to accepting Dwyer as an equal member of the human community, yet is so outraged by him that he wishes the man a "slow and painful death." These two things are incompatible. One cannot consider a person of equal value to all other persons and wish them a tortured end. The ethicist's dedication to the principle of equal regard does not appear to go all the way down, so that it is *felt* as well as *thought* (Pattern 14). If it did, he would first recognize Dwyer as a person, not a snake—and as a whole person, not only a murderer. Recognizing when our principles conflict with our feelings can be a first step to remediating our aversions; for the ethicist, this may allow him to reach out in common humanity to Dwyer and not only advocate for his listing as a candidate for transplant (as he did) but also wish for the transplant to be a success.

This discussion prompts another set of questions: Are there any *justifiable* "principled" aversions? If this story does not illustrate one, what set of circumstances might? By "principled" aversion, we mean an aversion based on an objective principle that *everyone* would be justified feeling, not one that is particular to individual persons, arising from their own past experiences and personal beliefs. With that definition, we are hard-pressed to imagine any justifiable "principled" aversions because we cannot imagine any principle that can justify *all of us* turning away from another person, refusing to see and treat that person as a human being—as the next section explains.

Everyone Is Worthy of Being Welcomed

We suspect that many readers are dismayed or outraged that we appear to advocate welcoming a person like Dwyer, who has done such awful things—and, more, to argue for being sufficiently open to him that we can desire his continued presence in the world. How can that be right or good? An "aversion" to someone like Dwyer is not just a matter of some distaste one may have toward those who break the law. Dwyer is a murderer, twice over, and one of his victims was a child. It's not even clear that he feels any remorse for his actions. How can we possibly argue for welcoming such a person?

We can argue for welcoming Dwyer—more, we can make the larger claim that *no one is unworthy of being welcomed*—because everything in this book has been pointing toward this truth. We welcome others as the *whole persons* they are in the moment. We see and respect the human being, the unique person they are. This does not require that we respect or condone things they have done. Rather, we set aside our assumptions and stereotypes, and our aversions, and look for characteristics that confirm their humanity and help us welcome them (see Pattern 15).

Bryan Stevenson, a tireless advocate for prisoners, writes: "Proximity has taught me some basic and humbling truths, including this vital lesson: Each of us is more than the worst thing we've ever done."[5] We have emphasized throughout the importance of proximity (see Pattern 4 for introduction of the idea), of overcoming distance between ourselves and the one we intend to welcome. The ethicist in the story had the opportunity to let his nearness to Dwyer in their one meeting teach him the same humbling truth that Stevenson learned. Seeing the "more" that Dwyer is could have opened the ethicist to the "more" that is in himself, to the possibility that he *could* genuinely welcome Dwyer, could want him to be in the world, recovering from a successful heart transplant and not dying the tortured death he envisioned for him. There is no one who is not worthy of these efforts, no human person who is not owed the obligation of welcome.

Protective Aversions and Being a Welcoming Person

Although everyone can be welcomed by someone, that someone may not be me, or you, at least not in the form of direct engagement. This point takes us to the work of discerning whether our reluctance to engage with someone, even our certainty that we should not engage, springs from a remediable aversion ("principled" or otherwise) or from a truly protective aversion, a circumstance of our individual experience that means we cannot and should not be expected to step forward in welcome toward this particular person.

What if the nurse assigned to care for the man awaiting a heart transplant realizes that he's the person who killed her sister and niece? Or maybe he's not the one who did it, but what he did mirrors the disaster that struck her own family. In such a case, the work required for the nurse to open herself in welcome to him may well exact far too high a cost, a cost neither she nor anyone else should expect her to pay.

But someone can personally welcome this man—pay attention to him, engage with him, desire to be in proximity to him. Why not another nurse without such a personal history? Why not the ethicist in the story? The question we each need to ask when we find ourselves resistant to opening and responding to someone else is this: "Is it me this time? This person has done truly reprehensible things (or has spouted truly evil ideas), but he is a human being and attention must be paid. Someone must do this; someone can do this. *Is it me?* Am I the one being called to welcome this person? *Why not me?*"

To return to the nurse who cannot directly and personally welcome the patient who has committed murder, what if she is committed to being a welcoming person? She can still be welcoming but in a way that keeps her safe: She can see that someone else personally welcomes him. She can maintain her *welcoming orientation*—as opposed to being so disturbed by his past behavior that she bars the door to his room or cuts off contact with anyone who agrees to care for him—while also acknowledging that, this time, she's not the one to do the direct welcoming (see Patterns 27 and 28 about setting limits and sharing responsibility).

If encounters with murderers seem too unusual to consider, think about a more common situation that seems to be at least as difficult. A person who just moved into the neighborhood is a known sex offender; everyone on the block knows all about it, no one wants to have anything to do with him, and some neighbors are conferring about what they can do to drive him away.

The universal obligation to be welcoming expects two things of us in this situation. First, it asks us to acknowledge that there may be some people who *should not* be expected to be welcoming to this new neighbor—someone, for example, who was sexually molested in childhood and cannot face an encounter of any sort with someone who has done that to others. Welcoming each other and ourselves means understanding when the cost is too high to bear.

Second, it asks us to remember that even rightly convicted sex offenders are worthy of being welcomed. Someone can be openly responsive to him; someone can offer welcome to this new neighbor. Here again, we must each ask ourselves the essential question, "*Is it me?* This person has done terrible things, but he is a human being and attention must be paid. Someone can welcome this person. Is it me? *Why not me?*"

This example about a new person moving into a neighborhood may evoke images and expectations of what "welcoming a person to the neighborhood" usually means that can get in the way of understanding what is required here. An ethics of welcome does not ask anyone to knock on the new neighbor's door with a casserole in hand, nor does it insist that he be immediately invited to a neighborhood picnic. But certain things are required. He cannot be shunned or ignored as if he does not exist. He cannot be merely tolerated. He cannot be reduced to the "label" of sex offender, any more than John Rembert can be reduced to the "case" of JR (see Pattern 2).

Specific actions that are possible and fitting will vary according to the persons and situations involved, but welcoming him always means being open enough to reconsider and respond rather than react. The *perspectives* of welcome require neighbors to recognize this newcomer as a member of the human community and, now, of their more local geographic community, and as a person about whom there is more to know. Engaging in the basic *practices* of welcome means acknowledging his presence by nodding to him and making eye contact; respecting him by using his name appropriately and appreciating what he has to offer, perhaps his fine gardening skills; and not allowing ourselves to accept as true the stories that our imaginations make up about him. If he is hurt in a ditch by the side of the road or his house catches fire, being welcoming means being there to offer help, to answer the call when it comes (Pattern 3).

In all of this discussion about taking the risk to be open and responsive to someone whose behavior has been appalling, even criminal, it must be clearly stated that there is nothing about being welcoming that overrides the commonsense importance of staying safe. Persons known to be potentially dangerous are not unworthy of welcome, but they should surely not be approached alone. Take someone with you, leave the door open, maintain an appropriate physical distance even as you try to overcome the relational space between the two of you with your words and gestures. *If the danger is acute, it is obviously not the time to offer welcome.* If the sex offender who has moved into your neighborhood is a pedophile (most sex offenders are not), protect all children in the area; be sure they are appropriately cautioned and constantly observed when the person is in the vicinity. There are some people who pose such a threat that they cannot remain free in communities, but wherever they are housed, including maximum security prisons, our welcome can extend there as well. They, too, should not live in isolation.

We have no way of knowing what it really costs anyone to be open to someone else. Even for those impediments that we label as potentially remediable aversions, there may be someone for whom overcoming that resistance would be expecting too much. This is yet another reason why nothing about this discussion should be heard as or linked with judgment, of others or of ourselves. This is not about declaring anyone guilty for refusing to welcome or even for being insufficiently welcoming. Even the ethicist in the story we cite—we don't know the rest of his story, only what has been written. The pursuit of a well-developed, ingrained disposition to be welcoming is not about finding fault with others or with ourselves. It is about wanting to get better at being open and responsive persons—and at creating and participating in a community in which welcoming each other is the norm—in ways that are safe and possible for us.

When we're faced with having to welcome someone we find repellent, we have to be honest with ourselves—that, too, is part of welcoming ourselves. We must be honest enough to distinguish between, on the one hand, a real incapacity, born from our own experience of life, that means we need to take care of ourselves and back away—it is not me, not this time—and, on the other hand, a reluctance to engage that arises from resistance to making the effort, understanding differently, and letting go of some comfortable but inadequately examined certainties.

When welcoming someone is particularly difficult, or even seems impossible, remember that everyone deserves to be welcomed by someone. Ask, "Is it me? Why not me?"

Notes

1 Arthur Miller, *Death of a Salesman*, in *The Portable Arthur Miller*, ed. Harold Clurman (Viking Press, New York, 1971), 50.
2 Ronald Munson, "Not More Equal," in *The Woman Who Decided to Die: Challenges and Choices at the Edges of Medicine* (Oxford University Press, New York, 2009), 103–17.
3 This is also currently the policy in the US. The Organ Procurement and Transplantation Network, which maintains the national registry for organ placement, holds that people who are incarcerated for committing crimes are not "sentenced by society to an additional punishment of an inability to receive consideration for medical services" and are "deemed worthy of equal treatment" in consideration of their candidacy for transplant. United Network for Organ Sharing (UNOS) ethics committee position statement regarding convicted

criminals and transplant evaluation, https://optn.transplant.hrsa.gov/professionals/by-topic/ethical-considerations/convicted-criminals-and-transplant-evaluation/, accessed February 20, 2025.

4 This characterization of tolerance and the points that follow draw deeply upon John R. Bowlin's thorough and indispensable discussion in *Tolerance among the Virtues* (Princeton University Press, Princeton, 2016).

5 Bryan Stevenson, *Just Mercy: A Story of Justice and Redemption* (One World, New York, 2015), 17–18.

27

Making Choices, Setting Limits

When the costs of welcoming another person are high—when what an ethics of welcome asks seems to be too much to expect of ourselves—we can make choices about our approaches and responses, setting limits as necessary while still maintaining a welcoming orientation.

In early 2018, one of us presented the story and welcome-oriented analysis of Dr. Wilson and Ms. Smythe's encounter (see Patterns 24 and 25) to a group of advanced medical students. She described how Ms. Smythe, an older White nursing home resident, when first meeting Dr. Wilson, the home's new medical director, blurted out that the physician was Black and then later in her medical appointment asked if she could choose a different doctor to be her primary care physician. The students were asked to consider whether Dr. Wilson had an obligation to help Ms. Smythe welcome her, and to notice that Dr. Wilson may have borne costs whichever course she took, whether she chose to deepen her welcoming efforts and risk receiving insulting or hateful comments in return, or to abandon such efforts and risk neglecting her professional commitments.

The students seemed taken aback by the depth of the obligation of welcome proposed and the breadth of its reach. Some of the students absolutely balked at the suggestion that Dr. Wilson may have had an obligation to help Ms. Smythe welcome her as her new doctor. One student said, forcefully and with more than a tinge of anger, that being a health professional did not mean she had to be a "welcome mat."

The students' comments were remarkably helpful to us as we continued to work on this book's project. Their resistance to reflecting on the broad scope of Dr. Wilson's obligations reminded us how radical this ethics of welcome is, how personal, how persistent (some might say relentless), and how demanding. We understood the student using the "welcome mat" expression to mean that she was not open to any approach to ethics that meant she would be trampled on and walked over, completely disregarded, and disrespected (see Pattern 21 about the fear of being manipulated). This is not what an ethics of welcome requires or how it was presented. But that's where her mind went, at least partly because we did not also explain (because we had not yet thought through) how particular personal boundaries can be appropriately set and honored within the boundless ethics of welcome required for human flourishing.

What's striking about the metaphor the student used is that a welcome mat is entirely passive. In sharp contrast, an ethics of welcome can be costly and demanding, but it is in no way passive. It is, in fact, *radically active*. It requires keenly active observation of what is happening around us and intensely active discernment about how we should respond, including, when appropriate, how we are to set limits when the costs of welcoming a particular person are too high. That is, it requires us to make choices—as opposed to having choices made for us—at every point.

Choosing to Set Limits

Consider a scenario we imagined in Pattern 26: a nurse discovers that a hospitalized patient to whom she has been assigned is the man who killed her sister and niece. She asks to be reassigned so that she may remain physically removed from this man. Although she is committed to being a welcoming person, she cannot summon the desire to be in the presence of this person, to make eye contact, to say his name, to go into his room, or, if she does go in, to stay there. She is not open to him; she does not want to be in his presence *at all*, to engage with him *in any way*, and this is unlikely to change, at least in the short term, perhaps ever. She cannot engage in welcoming practices with this patient because doing so would come at a cost she cannot reasonably bear. Engaging in welcoming actions in this situation could threaten her very self and violate her equal obligation to welcome herself. Indeed, it is difficult to imagine how she *could* welcome both him *and* herself, though we realize that some people do manage the unfathomable. This time it is not her (Patterns 8 and 26).

Her closed stance—the opposite of the open stance of welcome—toward this particular person at this time does not mean she is an unwelcoming person. As long as the limits she sets on her engagement, the boundaries she creates between herself and this other person, are appropriate (about which, more later), she has not done anything contrary to an ethics of welcome. Because even in such circumstances—when any one of us, out of consideration of high personal costs, deliberately assumes a closed stance toward someone and forgoes welcoming actions—we nevertheless can maintain a *welcoming orientation*. We can continue to believe that the other person deserves to be welcomed in the world. Even though we cannot be the ones at this time, to personally welcome them, we can nevertheless desire that others do so and place no impediments in their way.

This nurse/patient scenario is unusual and extreme. More typically, we face situations in which we can carry out fundamental welcoming practices, such as those identified in Part III, but also want to hold back from engaging more than seems called for. Sometimes we sincerely want to be in someone's presence, but not as much as they want to be with us—or what is needed or requested by the person we welcome is something we are unwilling to do.

> A woman has been caring as a lay minister for a member of her church who is experiencing a difficult time in her life. According to the norms of the program, the lay minister and care receiver meet regularly for an hour a week for as many weeks as needed. This care receiver can be unpleasant and challenging to be with, but the lay minister has been able to be positive and supportive of her during their visits. Early in the relationship they found they shared an interest in gardening, and the care receiver asked to see the lay minister's garden. The visit occurred, but the lay minister found the experience quite intrusive and exhausting.

Their regular weekly sessions resumed without difficulty; the lay minister found she could still offer support and attentive care in those short visits. But now the care receiver is once again hinting that she would love to spend more time in the lay minister's garden. The lay minister does not want to invite her there again given how troubling the first visit was. Does her obligation to be welcoming to her care receiver mean that she has to invite her anyway?

The answer is no. Her stance toward the care receiver is still one of welcome, of desire to engage and connect, to respect and care, to know her and accept her as she is, even to spend precious time with her, to be in proximity to her. There are many fitting ways to express and embody that open responsiveness. No specific way is mandated.

Even when we are being fully welcoming toward another person, the fitting response—what is good and right for the situation and the persons involved—can be a simple, limited interaction. To return to an example we often use, usually we can sincerely welcome a cashier at the grocery store without extending the interaction beyond checkout. Welcome does not blow up the normal parameters of particular kinds of encounters and the expected, useful boundaries that shape them. Welcoming someone does not mean we are not still in a customer-clerk, student-teacher, or patient-doctor relationship with them, subject to the norms and requirements of those settings. Even in the more personal and less constrained bonds of family and friendship, like the connection between the lay minister and the care receiver, being welcoming does not mean that we are required to meet all of someone's needs and desires, solve their problems, be with them as much as they might want, or the like.

The fundamental practices of welcome—for example, calling people by their names, imagining a different story—are open to choice in their details. Whether someone is called by their first name or an honorific, what different story is imagined are always particular and situational decisions, depending upon what is fitting for *both* persons. And, beyond the basic, obligatory practices of welcome, what else may be called for—among all the possible ways in which we can engage with someone and respond to their requests and needs—is a function of multiple factors. It may be entirely fitting, for example, for the lay minister to respond to the care receiver's hints for a return visit to the garden by instead pointing out a local garden show or sharing some of her daffodil bulbs. At times, it may be appropriate to say "no" or "I'm sorry, that's not possible," with or without an explanation. We can be open to others' needs without taking on responsibility for fulfilling them, a point considered further in the following pattern on sharing responsibility (Pattern 28).

Sometimes, then, the limits we set on our interactions with others are part of a fitting response within welcome, as they are for the lay minister who chooses not to invite the care receiver to her garden. At other times, the limits we set are on welcome itself, as is the case for the nurse in the hypothetical scenario—a choice to close the door and remain outside the presence of the other person, because we have determined that it is not wise for us personally to reach out in welcome.

Our actions or omissions in each instance may look similar; each sort of limit-setting may involve, for example, decisions that are protective of our time, resources, energy, or emotional investment. As a practical matter, we cannot constantly ask ourselves which sort of limits—*within* welcome or *on* welcome—we are setting for each encounter with each person.

On the other hand, sometimes the question *should* nag us. At times, it should be asked because the answer may reveal a lack of openness toward someone, a closed stance that we have adopted without adequate attention and intention and that is not justified by the risk of exceptionally high personal costs. That is, we may think we're setting reasonable limits within welcome, when in fact we are refusing to welcome at all. Recognizing when this is the case can prompt us to think again about the choices we have made and to reconsider what we know or think we know of the other person and our relationship with them.

Blanket Refusals to Welcome

Each of the situations we present—Dr. Wilson and Ms. Smythe, the nurse and her assigned patient, the lay minister and the care receiver—involves people making decisions about welcoming a particular other person. At times, however, it is tempting to make such decisions about *categories* of people.

Let's return to the medical students who were not happy with the suggestion that Dr. Wilson may have had an obligation to help Ms. Smythe welcome her as her new doctor. The intensity of emotion with which the student made the "welcome mat" comment suggested that she was reacting to something other than, or in addition to, the story itself, reminding us that, as with many situations described in this book, we don't always know the entire context in which they take place.

> The class session took place in the spring of 2018, following the nationally reported White supremacy events that took place in Charlottesville during the summer of 2017—the July march of the Ku Klux Klan and the much larger August 12th Unite the Right rally that drew White supremacists from around the country and left one counter-protester dead and many injured. The night before the Unite the Right rally, White supremacists carried lit torches on the treasured Lawn of the University of Virginia and menacingly surrounded students who stood with arms linked around a central statue of Thomas Jefferson.
>
> When the medical students in the seminar protested the radical obligations associated with an ethics of welcome, they may have been still raw from these experiences. The University health system had also seen an uptick in discriminatory and bigoted remarks (as did many health systems and society in general) during the students' years in medical school. They may have observed or been more directly involved in situations in which patients had insulted and demanded not to be treated by doctors, nurses, or students of a particular skin color or with a foreign-sounding accent or displaying a certain symbol of faith. Such demands were becoming more common and more insistent (see Pattern 29 for discussion of the health system's response). Plus, the student making the "welcome mat" comment was female. Female medical students have also long been recipients of comments implying they are less competent than their male counterparts and subjected to inappropriate comments about their appearance or attractiveness.

Considering this context, it was understandable for this student and others to express consternation upon being asked or expected to be welcoming toward every single person they encountered. How could they welcome people like the torchbearers, the Klan members, and other overt bigots who might be their patients?

We have approached this complex question in many different ways in this book, asserting that a person can be welcomed without approving all their behaviors and that what we know, or think we know, about a person is not all there is to know. (We have suggested, for example, that Ms. Smythe's terse remark does not tell us whether she bore animosity toward either Dr. Wilson or Black health professionals generally.) And for practitioners, there may be professional obligations not only to see that patients receive appropriate care but also, in doing so, to go through the motions of welcome even when feeling otherwise (Pattern 14).

We each have to figure out for ourselves when we cannot personally engage in some or any welcoming actions toward another, such as one of the overtly bigoted patients the students were imagining being asked to take care of. We must evaluate our own tolerance for risk, assess our own costs, and make our own decisions in each situation about whether the risks are too high and the potential costs too much to bear. If we judge the costs to ourselves to be too high, we can set limits to our engagement. And there is nothing about an ethics of welcome that says we cannot directly call out racist or other noxious behaviors. But it does insist that our decisions must be based on the actual person before us, not on the stereotype or category we have assigned to that person (Pattern 13).

An ethics of welcome does not ask or expect anyone to be a welcome mat. It asks that we make intentional choices, specific to individual persons and specific encounters, about how (and sometimes if) we are to open ourselves to and engage with this particular person. It does not permit a blanket rejection of a category of persons on the basis of prejudgments and stereotyping. This would be counter to the perspectives of welcome (Part II) and would undermine our efforts to maintain a welcoming orientation.

Limiting Welcome While Maintaining a Welcoming Orientation

A welcoming orientation is a settled disposition or virtue—a way of being in the world—that embodies a commitment to being a welcoming person and understands capacious welcome to be essential for human flourishing. It includes both the view that all persons, at all times, are capable and deserving of being welcomed (by someone) and the desire that they be so welcomed.

The obligation to maintain a welcoming orientation helps identify limits that can appropriately be set at those unusual times when we determine that the costs of being open and responsive to a particular person are too high for us to bear, for those times when we have closed the door. Moreover, whether limits are set on welcome or within welcome, their scope, form, and duration should be carefully fitted to the situation at hand. We offer here some general rules of thumb. They are neither exhaustive nor finely tuned.

Limits on welcome should be set only as necessary. We can set limits on welcome in ways required to protect ourselves from costs we have determined to be unacceptably high, but only what is needed for that purpose, not more. The justification for the limits—the need for self-preservation and the obligation to welcome oneself—is the guiding principle.

For example, in Pattern 25, we consider whether the physician-narrator in the poem by Danny Abse could have remained both true to himself *and* welcoming by directly responding to a patient who spewed prejudicial venom, insisting that he stop his offensive speech. We also noted that if the patient did not desist and instead continued on as before, the doctor would not be wrong to end the encounter (unless the patient needed immediate, urgent care). Protecting himself from harm might require the doctor, in his judgment, to set this limit on engagement. However, suppose that the patient later returns to apologize and offer some explanation for his offensive behavior. The doctor's appropriately self-protective move to limit engagement does not prevent him from considering this further information—from reconsidering the patient (Pattern 15)—with the possibility that he could once again offer welcome.

Setting limits does not include or allow engaging in unwelcoming practices. Deciding not to engage in welcoming practices does not mean that practices in direct opposition to welcoming practices are acceptable. It would not be appropriate, for example, to relish stereotyping another person, to bring a hidden agenda to a meeting with them, or to deliberately misuse their name. Engaging in unwelcoming practices is incompatible with a welcoming orientation.

Limits are set for ourselves, not for others. Deciding that one cannot personally welcome someone does not mean that it is acceptable to prevent others from doing so. Everyone can be welcomed by someone (see Pattern 26). I may find myself unable to "step into the room" with a particular person, but I must not then bar the door to others who *can* enter. The nurse who cannot reasonably be expected to welcome the man who killed her sister and niece must not stand in the way of having another nurse be assigned to him or shun those who can offer him care. Limits surround the welcoming person like a protective bubble; they do not create a barrier around the other person.

Other ethical obligations remain. Setting limits on or within welcome does not cancel the call of other ethical requirements, such as duties to be fair and honest or to fulfill contractual or professional obligations. Welcome is the *primary* obligation, not the only obligation; the *primary* perspective, not the only perspective; the *primary* virtue, not the only virtue. Recall that the students who observed Dr. Wilson's and Ms. Smythe's encounter (Pattern 24) wondered whether, were they in the doctor's shoes, they would have immediately terminated the visit; one even wondered whether she would have been tempted not to prescribe pain medication. Their lack of openness toward Ms. Smythe is troubling and likely unjustifiable under an ethics of welcome but, regardless of the limits they may set on welcoming her, a decision to abandon her or refuse to provide appropriate treatment would be an independent and significant ethical lapse.

Set limits as needed within *welcome in open, responsive ways that are fitting for you and for the other person. Set limits on welcome only when absolutely necessary because of unacceptably high costs, and be willing to periodically reevaluate the scope of those limits. Always maintain a welcoming orientation.*

28

Sharing the Responsibility

Responsibility to welcome others in the human community belongs to everyone and should be shared. Sharing the responsibility for welcome is essential for human flourishing.

In Pattern 26, we offer the question "Is it me?" as one for us all to ask ourselves when we feel reluctant or unable to welcome some person. If our carefully considered answer is, "This time, it's not me," there remains one more question to ask as we limit our welcoming engagement: *"If not me, then who?"* We can and should look to others to share the human responsibility to welcome a person we ourselves cannot fully welcome. Moreover, even in the more common situation when we are able to engage in welcoming actions, it is equally appropriate to ask, *"Who, in addition to me?"* Determining who else can welcome another and facilitating and supporting their welcoming efforts are vital components of the work of welcome.

Margaret has frequently given talks to medical audiences about the importance of physicians being open and responsive to their patients, listening to their stories and receiving the expression, however subtle, of their deepest questions and concerns, including the spiritual ones. Many times, someone in the audience, during the Q&A part of the presentation, would gently remind her that there is a team, one that includes nurses, social workers, chaplains, and others. These things need doing, but the doctor is not the only one available or, in some cases, best equipped to do them. Eventually, Margaret learned to incorporate that vital point about shared responsibility into her talks.

We imagine all of us have needed such a reminder from time to time, in going about various aspects of our lives—completing a project at work, hosting a party, caring for a sick loved one—because nearly always there *are* others who are already working toward the same goal or who are ready to step in. The recognition that we are part of a team that shares the responsibility of welcome enables us to engage in our own welcoming practices, determine fitting responses within welcome, and set limits when necessary.

We expand this concept of teamwork and sharing responsibility in order to integrate within it the related ideal of "nested welcome," in which we are each nested within and supported by informal, small, self-forming welcoming groups that are themselves nested within larger welcoming institutions, which in turn are nested within wider welcoming communities. This concept is inspired by the work of Eva Feder Kittay, an American feminist philosopher working within an ethics of care, who developed the related model of "nested dependencies."[1] Kittay was concerned about who takes care of "dependency workers"—people whose work involves caring for those whose lives are dependent on such care—especially ones who are not paid to do it, like mothers of dependent children or caregivers of family members with disabilities. Recognizing that there usually cannot be reciprocity in such relationships, she pointed out that the dependency worker herself depends upon others recognizing and fulfilling their obligations to support her. "The dependency worker is entitled not to reciprocity from the charge herself, but to a relationship that sustains her as she sustains her charge" (68). This entitlement grounds a "public ethic of care" in which the larger society is obligated "to support the dependency relationship and the individuals that constitute it" (128).

This nesting within nesting creates redundancies that protect against our ethical failings at various levels, as individuals or in groups. We illustrate this notion by way of a story shared with us by a graduate student in social work. The student was working as an intern with a nonprofit organization that brings community resources into public schools to help students stay in school and engaged.

> An elementary school student with epilepsy had a seizure at school. School administrators, along with the school nurse and a Spanish translator, met several times with the family, for whom English was a new language, to ensure that the child saw a neurologist and to explain that the parents needed to provide written consent for the school to administer emergency

medication if needed. The parents failed to provide the medication and necessary consent, and the school nurse intended to call the state's child protective services agency to report the parents for medical neglect.

Upon learning this, the community support group working with the school requested that another meeting be held with the parents before a report was made to the state agency. The following day the parents arrived on time at the school for the meeting. The meeting was translated in Spanish and English by one of the support group's employees who also had a daughter with a seizure disorder. The parents agreed with the school's plan for administering emergency medication. They asked questions about the needed forms and explained that their daughter had seen a neurologist and been prescribed an emergency seizure medication, but that it was very expensive, and they did not have insurance to cover it. The community support group's employee offered to help the family enroll in a program that provides free medications to those in need. The parents returned to the school a second time that day with all the items they were told to bring to enroll in the program.

For us, this is a story of nested welcome. The parents, the school, the community support group, the state agency, the program that provides free medications to those who cannot afford them, even the courts, if they had had to be engaged—all of these, in an ideal world, are committed to meeting the needs of the child. But that commitment alone is not enough. Indeed, it is easy to imagine a counter-scenario in which the school carries out its commitment by reporting the parents. Intrusive home inspections, mandated doctors' appointments, court hearings, and worse follow, all experienced by the parents and child as punitive and bewildering—a swirl intensified by cultural and language differences—and no one, at the end of the day, is better off.

Instead, when those involved welcomed each other in their shared goal of caring for the child, they could more readily ensure that her needs were appropriately met. The redundancies of care—not simply of a moral obligation to safeguard the well-being of the child, but *redundancies of welcoming engagement*—worked.

Let's back up to where things stood before the meeting, before the work of nested welcome showed results. School personnel were about to refer the parents to the state agency. Many factors likely contributed to this plan, including problems in communication, bureaucratic requirements, the daily pressures of juggling the needs of a large number of students and staff, perhaps even stereotyping. They culminated in the school's intention to *deflect* responsibility for the child's well-being to the state agency.

When the community support group stepped in, serving as a welcoming nest around the child, the parents, and the school staff members, the school was able to *share* its responsibility. The parents could demonstrate their care for their child and receive the assistance they needed. The school staff members could gain a truer understanding of the parents and their situation and have their many concerns resolved. Ideally, the school's productive collaboration with the community support group would inform its future actions with this and other families.

In this story, the focus is primarily on how the redundancies of nested welcome and shared responsibility benefit the ones being welcomed. Now we turn to how nested welcome aids the one who wishes to welcome. As we wrestle with the challenges of fulfilling our own individual responsibilities well, we should be able to rely on the responsibility of the rest of society, often through communities and organizations, to take care of us. *Knowing that we are welcomed is what makes it possible for us to be welcoming.* David Barnard, an expert in the ethical, spiritual, and psychological dimensions of illness and healing, put it this way: "The conviction that we are 'held,' in an ultimate sense, validates every particular embrace, and finally permits every letting go."[2] Barnard is speaking about transcendent or divine support, but the same point applies to the essential support and care we require from each other in order to go about the work of welcome.

Let us return briefly to the story of Dr. Wilson, the Black physician, and Ms. Smythe, the White patient who blurted out that Dr. Wilson was Black (Pattern 24). An ethics of welcome calls on Dr. Wilson to try to help Ms. Smythe welcome her, but it also calls on the nursing home, health system, and society at large to fully welcome Dr. Wilson. Dr. Wilson's apparent difficulty in going a step further in trying to establish a relationship with Ms. Smythe may well be explainable by her own long-standing experience and expectation of not being welcomed as a physician or even as a person more generally in a predominantly White society. The medical students who witnessed that encounter in real time, as well as those who reacted passionately to its retelling several years later (Pattern 27), may also be familiar with feeling unwelcome.

When we presented the story of Dr. Wilson and Ms. Smythe to medical students some years later, their indignant reaction—captured in "I am not a welcome mat!"—seemed to be influenced by the rising number of patients who refused to be cared for by certain healthcare professionals on account of their race, ethnicity, or religion (see the discussion in Pattern 27). Of interest for the subject of this pattern is how the university health system and medical school began to address what was, in fact, a long-standing problem. In the aftermath of the Unite the Right Rally, institutional leaders expressly recognized the problem for what it was. It was not simply that certain practitioners and students were, and long had been, on the receiving end of bigoted behaviors; it was that, though these reprehensible behaviors were usually observed by others, nothing was routinely done about them. Occasionally, someone spoke up either to correct the patient or, more often, to offer words of support to their colleague later and out of earshot of the patient. But there were no explicit expectations of the observer, even if that person had greater power or authority within the system than the person targeted (e.g., an attending physician or nurse manager observing a resident doctor or staff nurse being abused, or a resident or nurse observing the same of a medical or nursing student). Nothing was expected of the institutional community in response to overt, demeaning, and hurtful bigotry. The responsibility for dealing with the situation, shamefully, was left to the one who had been attacked.

In attempts to change that, the university health system adopted and prominently posted statements about the responsibilities of patients not to reject caregivers on the basis of characteristics that we typically understand as protected against discrimination such as race, religion, and ethnicity. Concerted efforts were made to train everyone within the organization to be prepared for these situations, to address a patient's derogatory statements directly by standing up for the targeted person, and to examine and, in most cases, reject a patient's bigoted demand for a different provider.[3] By making these changes, the health system and its professional schools welcomed their employees, faculty, students, and trainees, holding them within a nest of welcome so that those workers could then step out confidently in welcome toward all their patients and colleagues, however troublesome.

Shared responsibility for welcome characterizes a flourishing human community. Much of what follows from this observation is obvious and needn't be belabored: Sometimes the most fitting response in welcome is to connect the one we are welcoming to other people. When we need to set a limit on our welcoming engagement, we may also have a responsibility to ensure that someone else will step in. And sometimes we need to be the one to notice that someone else cannot or should not be expected to personally welcome a particular person, and then to step up and step in ourselves to provide the needed welcome—of both persons. Responsible ways to deal with recognized responsibilities include not only taking them on and fulfilling them but also— and of equal importance—assigning them to or sharing them with others.[4]

Build nests. Allow and encourage others to join in your welcoming actions. See that those expected to be welcoming (all of us) are also experiencing welcome and the support it gives. Be aware of or ask for your own needed support.

Notes

1. Eva Feder Kittay, *Love's Labor: Essays on Women, Equality, and Dependency* (Routledge, New York, 1999), 107.
2. David Barnard, "Religion and Medicine: A Meditation on Lines by A.J. Heschel," *Soundings* 68 (1985): 443–65, at 463.
3. This last issue—whether it is ethical ever to accede to a patient's demand for a different caregiver on account of their race or ethnic background—is complicated. One multidisciplinary group of scholars studying the issue asserts that "requests for an ethnically or racially concordant physician may be ethically appropriate in certain cases." Paul-Emile Kimani, Alexander K. Smith, Bernard Lo, and Alicia Fernandez, "Dealing with Racist Patients," *New England Journal of Medicine* 374, no. 8 (2016): 708–11. They give examples based on religion, such as Muslim women requesting female physicians, and on deep-seated distrust of providers,

as may justifiably be experienced by African Americans based on a long history of discrimination within health care. Requests for reassignment of care that are simply bigoted, however, are generally not deserving of accommodation, although in rare cases they might merit consideration, such as when a patient is a "veteran with post-traumatic stress disorder who refuses treatment from a clinician of the same ethnic background as former enemy combatants."

4 See Margaret Urban Walker's discussion of the "marvelously intricate" practices of responsibility in *Moral Understandings: A Feminist Study in Ethics*, 2nd ed. (Oxford University Press, New York, 2007), 100.

29

A Fundamental View of the World

Wherever and whyever people gather, whether in the formal structures of an institution, by happenstance of geographical location, or out of a common interest or a shared goal, they take on group responsibilities to be welcoming.

Altogether, the patterns presented in this book offer "a fundamental view of the world," of the desirable world that results from each of us fulfilling our obligations to be welcoming. We borrow this expression and its expansive meaning from *A Pattern Language*, the work on architecture and liveability mentioned in this book's Introduction. What the architects of *A Pattern Language* meant by "a fundamental view of the world" was that none of the patterns they presented was isolated, and no aspect of the built environment was too small or too large to consider, alone or in combination. If you build a smaller thing, it will be influenced by and in turn influence a larger thing and become a part of it. They explained:

> This is a fundamental view of the world. It says that when you build a thing you cannot merely build that thing in isolation, but must also repair the world around it, and within it, so that the larger world at that one place becomes more coherent, and more whole; and the thing which you make takes its place in the web of nature, as you make it.[1]

In *A Pattern Language*, "the thing which you make"—a sheltering roof or town square—must be built in a way to "repair the world around it, and within it," so that the place where it is located becomes "more coherent, and more whole." In an ethics of welcome, the things we do—call people by their names, let people tell us who they are, invite the other person into our world—create a livable space of another kind, one in which each person in an encounter can be appreciated and valued, where everyone can be at home. That space always connects, in ways obvious and subtle, to the larger world around it. The relationships that we facilitate or build through welcome are acts of making and acts of repairing, changing not only ourselves and those whom we encounter but also, inevitably, others around the people with whom we are engaged. These rippling effects make human life in that place, in the communities and society thereby created, more habitable, more welcoming, more coherent, more whole.

In the geographical and political communities in which we live—neighborhoods, towns, counties, states—countless decisions, large and small, are made that determine their liveability: zoning laws, systems of policing and justice, taxation rules, protections for voting rights, funding for and attention to childcare and schools, whether and where we create green spaces, parks, and playgrounds, where we put roads and crosswalks, the amount and kind of public art that is funded, the hours libraries are open, and so on. When made well, these decisions manifest welcome by showing respect and equal regard for all, recognizing everyone as "worthy," and worthy to the same degree. Everyone fits in; each person is included (or, at least no one is intentionally excluded) in the space, now community-wide, that welcome creates.

Other types of communities can be formed by shared interests, like clubs or teams; by shared affiliations, like cultural, religious, and ethnic associations; and by shared pursuits, like institutions in which we work and with which we interact. Such groups, like society more generally, are shaped by multiple decisions that reflect how the persons within them and those whom they affect or with whom they interact are valued and welcomed.

Therefore, although in most of this book we describe encounters, relationships, and responsibilities between two people, in this pattern we claim that groups *as groups* also have obligations to be welcoming and that their engagement in practices of welcome is essential to building a livable, coherent world for us all. We first explain why the obligation to be welcoming applies to groups as well as to individual persons. To do so, we narrow our focus to those groupings that are formal institutions (companies, schools and colleges, hospitals, libraries, factories, theaters, fitness centers, and so on) because of their prominence in modern society, their clear and often obligatory pursuit of other goals (like creating a product, making a profit, or keeping the doors open), and their seemingly impersonal nature.

We then take note of the many disparate and often seemingly small decisions that well-intentioned people, individually and collectively, make within organizations that build and foster community or undercut and neglect it. Being welcoming is a constant and demanding moral commitment. Every policy, practice, and decision that affects people has ethical significance. You may recognize this idea from our Introduction, where we first assert, radically, that the obligation of welcome applies to every encounter, every time. Everything matters. Nothing takes place in isolation.

Why Institutions Have Obligations to Be Welcoming and Why It Matters

This section focuses on institutions, but keep in mind that the understanding of welcome and its obligations expressed here applies in similar ways to all formal and informal associations of people. It may be puzzling to hear that institutions—which often are characterized as cold (or at least detached), impersonal, efficient, businesslike, singularly focused, with lives of their own separate from the people who work within them—have an *obligation* to be welcoming. It is perhaps easier to appreciate that institutional policies, practices, and norms can be more or less open and responsive to their workers, customers and clients, and the general public, and that institutions can encourage or inhibit welcoming practices by the persons who work in them and those with whom they interact.

Elsewhere in the book, we present positive examples of welcoming practices adopted by institutions: hospitals that facilitated video visitation by family members during the Covid-19 pandemic when in-person hospital visitation was not allowed (Pattern 4); an assisted living facility that replaced rigid diet regimens, schedules, and "truth-telling" with more flexible practices to meet the needs and desires of residents with dementia (Pattern 23). These stories involved health care institutions, but similar stories could be offered about the practices of any sort of organization or workplace. That institutions *can* do these things is clear; why *must* they?

The answer is both obvious and simple. Institutions have obligations to be welcoming *because they are made up of people making decisions that affect other people.* If an ethics of welcome calls on each of us to be welcoming and responsible in every aspect of our lives, then that call obviously includes the decisions we make and the activities we perform at work, in the organizations in which we volunteer, in the groups where we gather, and in the polities of which we are a part. The policies, norms, practices, and culture of an institution are never established by that impersonal organization; they are established by persons working within it.

To be clear, we are not asserting that any institution's *primary* obligation is to be welcoming in the same way that we claim the primary ethical obligation of individual persons is to be welcoming. Indeed, American corporate law generally holds that the primary responsibility of a for-profit company is to financially benefit its shareholders; they are the ones, some would say the only ones, who count. (In recent decades, "stakeholder theory" has provided a strong counterpoint within business ethics to that traditionally recognized singular pursuit; stakeholder theory holds that obligations are also owed to employees, suppliers, local geographic communities, and other constituencies.[2]) Nonprofit corporations are established to pursue particularly defined missions such as to provide health care, educate children, settle refugees, help veterans, or create places of worship. Less loosely organized associations, such as book clubs and running groups, are likewise formed for various discrete purposes.

What we *are* saying is that if the people who work in, volunteer with, join, or otherwise have a voice in these organizations are obligated to be welcoming—as they are—then, both individually and collectively, they must critically evaluate the institution's practices through the lens of welcome. When empowered to make or contribute to decisions in pursuit of the institution's goals, they should consider whether and how the institution's actions are or are not welcoming, including whether those actions encourage or impede their own and others' individual efforts to be welcoming. In doing so, we believe, they also often promote the more particular goals of the organization.

We have observed many institutional endeavors with this double action, where intentionally engaging in welcoming actions allows other good ends of the organization to be achieved. Consider, for example, the following:

> Several years ago, the director of our institution's research ethics board noticed that the community members on the board were mostly silent in meetings. She and others had taken care to express words of welcome and clear appreciation for their service, but they still appeared reluctant to speak up.
>
> For a community member, board meetings can be intimidating. The research proposals that are reviewed are lengthy, dense, and highly scientific. Nearly all the other board members come from the institution and are highly educated experts like physicians, pharmacologists, statisticians. Plus, everyone except the community member is in an environment familiar to them, a conference room on campus; they are at home. The community members' relative silence was understandable, even predictable.
>
> The director tried a new approach. She gave community members the task of analyzing the consent forms that the subjects of a proposed research study would sign in order to participate, and reporting their findings to the board. They were, after all, uniquely positioned to consider the forms and proposed studies from the perspective of a potential research subject who knows little about medical research and nothing about the researchers' reputations. With this new role, they no longer had to discern when and whether to speak up or wonder if their contributions had value because they now had a place on the meeting's agenda.

Now, why is this an example of welcome? One could say this was just a means to satisfy a regulatory requirement for input from nonscientists outside the organization. Yes and no. Having community members on the board is required, but the regulations do not, cannot dictate that their presence be desired or useful. The spirit of the regulations may call for meaningful input from community members, but mere tokenism is permitted.

With their new initiative, the ethics board leadership showed they did in fact desire the community members' presence—the essential meaning of welcome—and recognized what they had to offer. Whether the director was motivated by the intended purpose of the regulations to include community voices, by her own welcoming orientation, or—what we suspect is most likely—by some combination of the two, does not need untangling, since these intentions work hand in hand.

These good efforts, we are sorry to say, were abandoned (temporarily, one hopes) after that director retired. Under new leadership, longtime community members left the board, and the requirement for "community" representation was satisfied only technically—the need for nonscientist members was met by appointing persons from other disciplines in the institution, and the need for nonaffiliated members was met by appointing retired scientists. The past director's commitment to meaningful community involvement apparently had not received the recognition and support from other board members and from institutional leaders above her necessary for these welcoming practices to continue beyond her tenure.

To become lasting and embedded enough to be considered an *institutional* practice, rather than a single person's way of doing things, a practice must receive a collective endorsement from others within the institution. Only then can the practice endure, deepen, and be integrated into the institution's culture in a way that can affect or "repair" the wider organizational environment and beyond. One can imagine a counterfactual in which the continued robust welcome of community members on the research ethics board led to greater community involvement in other aspects of the health system's work. Such a development would expand the possibilities of shared responsibility for the community's health needs and create the sort of "nested welcome" that would enhance the institution's work in all sorts of ways (see Pattern 28).

Consider, as a contrasting example, the supportive, welcoming institutional response given to the problematic situation presented in Pattern 20, in which the hidden agenda of representatives of an organ procurement organization (OPO) caused consternation among the nurses in an intensive care unit.

> The ICU nurses felt they could not protect their patients' families from less than forthright interactions with the OPO representatives who were spending time with family members in order to be positioned, at the right

time, to obtain consent for organ donation. Some nurses also felt pressured to obscure the true purpose of the OPO representatives' presence (OPO representatives often provide a script for nurses to use to introduce them to a family simply as "someone who assists with end-of-life decisions"). The nurses were troubled enough to report to higher administration their apprehensions about the OPO's engagement with patients' families. They insisted that although organ donation is a worthy goal, efforts to secure donation should not override the primary goal of respecting and caring for the dying patient and their family, which required, among other things, honest communication.

Here's how the hospital responded: First, the nurses' voices were welcomed; persons in administrative roles with decision-making influence or power *listened* to their concerns. The often more powerful voices of the transplant surgeons, who did not at first appreciate some of the nuances of the situation, were not allowed to drown them out. The nurses' understanding of what was most important (truth-telling and loyalty to the patient) was welcomed although it differed from that of the OPO (which prioritized increasing the supply of organs without harm to others).

Second, the administrators *accepted responsibility* for addressing these concerns, as opposed to brushing them aside simply as "the way things are done" or as an unavoidable tension created by competing goals.

Third, they asked, "*How can we do this better?*" and involved both the nurses and OPO representatives and supervisors in answering that question. That is, rather than drawing battle lines, they brought people together. Over several months, numerous substantive and lasting changes were made that clarified the role of OPO representatives with patients' families and satisfied the concerns of the nurses.

The new procedures were a significant improvement in transparency, openness, and responsiveness. Because they were developed through a collaborative process that welcomed all involved in the situation, they became integrated into the fabric of the institution (unlike the temporary changes in the research ethics board). It is reasonable to surmise that the positive experience and outcome of this process, for all participants, encouraged other such welcoming collaborations, grounded in careful listening, acceptance of responsibility, and optimistic curiosity.

The Many Decisions Made by Institutions: Acts and Omissions

Myriad decisions are made each day that determine how welcoming an institution is, although sometimes those decisions are not consciously understood by anyone either to be ethical decisions or to have anything to do with welcome. Consider, for example, the way people are received at hospitals. The first person a patient entering a hospital's emergency department often sees or interacts with is a security guard. The second person is usually the one who asks for their insurance card. When a person is admitted to the hospital, one of the first questions they will be asked in the admissions process, with bureaucratic efficiency and no matter their medical condition or emotional state, is whether they have an advance directive with their end-of-life instructions documented. (Perhaps the hospital near you is different, but this is pretty much what you will encounter in ours and others we have visited.) None of these practices, even if necessary in some form and at some time, is likely to be experienced as welcoming, and each can even be seen as contrary to the therapeutic purposes of the institution adopting them. How is it that they come to be and remain in place?

Although practices like these may seem to have come about almost naturally, each is the result of a *decision*, a *choice* made by some person or group of persons about how best to run a hospital. Where should the security guard stand—here, here, or here? Which staff person at which point of encounter should be assigned to carry out the federal mandate to ask about advance directives? Unwelcoming environments encountered by incoming patients do not arise accidentally. Institutions adopt policies that create these environments and interfere with or obstruct their workers' efforts to be welcoming.

In other instances, particularly in this matter of working environments, it can be less clear that any actual choices have been made that contribute to an unwelcoming situation. Sometimes we are just neglectful, failing to notice or take seriously a problem that needs fixing. The decisions that together form unwelcoming environments or cultures may each seem so small and incremental as to be almost unnoticeable, though they can have an impact as significant as that of an overt and agonizingly debated choice. It may be only in retrospect that we can recognize judgments we have made that have brought us to where we are.

Consider the institutional response described in Pattern 27: During a period of heightened local and national White supremacist activity, leaders in our health system recognized that the institution needed to do more to support hospital staff and trainees who were vulnerable to being targeted by bigoted patients. This may seem to be an example of an institution promptly responding to a problem once brought to its leaders' attention. But this was by no means a new phenomenon, even if the increased frequency and intensity of the incidents made it harder to ignore. Similar acts of rejection and hateful rhetoric had long been directed at members of vulnerable groups in this hospital setting, as is surely the case elsewhere. The institution's corrective move was a good one—adopting policies and pursuing interventions to make workers feel welcomed and supported so that they, in turn, can be more welcoming to their patients, including the bigoted ones. But this positive outcome also reveals, by stark contrast, that earlier mistaken judgments, blindnesses, and failures to act by persons at all levels of responsibility in the institution had contributed significantly to a painfully unwelcoming environment for some.

In this instance, it was long-standing omissions in the hospital's policies—apparent failures to decide—that contributed to the unwelcoming situation; correction required the adoption of new strategies. In some of the previous examples (like the placement of the hospital security guard and the script the OPO gave to nurses), it was existing policies—overt decisions—that interfered with welcome; correction required that they be changed or scrapped altogether. Is there a moral difference between institutional *acts* and *omissions* that contribute to creating an unwelcoming environment? We doubt there is. In either case, decisions—including the decision not to see, not to question, not to decide—are being made by people. And what may look like an excusable failure to notice a problem is often the result of our choosing to look away, to pay attention elsewhere. *We are always either practicing welcoming or practicing its opposite* (Pattern 14), and that is as true of institutional decision-makers as it is of each of us individually.

This discussion of the obligations of welcome for institutions shows what welcome looks and acts like and can accomplish in all other sorts of human communities, and demonstrates the ways in which individual practices of welcome interact with, influence, and are influenced by the welcoming practices of groups of all sizes, from the smallest to the largest groupings. The practices that enabled the hospital in one of our examples to respond well to a group of troubled nurses can help us all, in each of the overlapping communities of which we are a part, to make real this fundamental view of a livable, welcoming world. Building welcoming communities, making our world coherent and whole, asks of us that we listen attentively to each other, that we accept our responsibilities, individually and as groups, and that we ask ourselves, over and over again, "How can we do this better?" and find our answers together.

Build welcoming communities at work, in your neighborhood, among people with whom you share particular interests. Invite others to join. Learn to spot when group practices, whether acts or omissions, contribute to unwelcoming environments. Work to change them.

Notes

1 Alexander et al., *A Pattern Language*, xiii.
2 See, for example, the work of R. Edward Freeman, including *Strategic Management: A Stakeholder Approach* (Cambridge University Press, New York, 2010).

30

Step into the Welcoming World

In a book of autobiographical reflections, Thomas Merton—writer, scholar, mystic, social activist, monk—describes a revelatory moment:

> In Louisville, at the corner of Fourth and Walnut, in the center of the shopping district, I was suddenly overwhelmed with the realization that I loved all these people, that they were mine and I theirs, that we could not be alien to one another even though we were total strangers. It was like waking from a dream of separateness . . .
>
> Then it was as if I suddenly saw the secret beauty of their hearts . . . If only they could all see themselves as they really are. If only we could see each other that way all the time. There would be no more war, no more hatred, no more cruelty, no more greed.[1]

There is now a historical marker at the corner of Fourth and Walnut in Louisville, Kentucky, to honor Merton's epiphany there (maybe the only such marker erected in recognition of a spiritual experience). It was presented to the city by the Thomas Merton Foundation, but whatever governmental group then authorized its prominent display seems to have thought that Merton's realization was worth repeating as a vision, whether accurate or aspirational, or both, of their community.

What a vision it is: a fundamental view of the world and of human beings that mirrors the view that is the rationale and theme of this book, of this ethics of welcome. A welcoming orientation—a desire to be in the presence of the persons we encounter and a settled disposition of open responsiveness toward them—nurtures and acts on this essential realization: we *cannot* "be alien to one another." With that insight, we can glimpse the "secret beauty" at the heart of each of us that defines who we human beings really are, even given the evils we do and the evils done in our name. None of us is unworthy of being welcomed; none of us is unworthy of being loved. "If only we could see each other that way all the time."

Merton's words connect the concept of welcoming developed in this book to age-old traditions of moral and spiritual thought, both religious and humanist, that use the language of love to describe our interconnectedness and our obligations and responsibilities to each other. Indeed, many of you may understand and expand upon ideas in the book through the lens of love. The similarities are evident; we allude to them in our Introduction. But we offer the "new" language of welcome because it is so much clearer about what is being asked of us, because it moves us to action, and because being welcoming is a concrete, graspable *practice*—or, perhaps better, a group of practices—that we can work on and get better at, that we can adopt and adapt to each new encounter as well as to each long-standing relationship.

The perspectives and practices of welcome, described at length in this book, thus give needed substance to the otherwise unspecified call to love one another. They explicate and illuminate what open responsiveness to another person entails and where it can take us. But what actually happens in a welcoming encounter is not dictated with any specificity by an ethics of welcome. Rather, it is determined by who the actors are, what the circumstances of the encounter may be, what needs are revealed, and what fitting responses are called for. Every welcoming encounter is like every other in that they are moments of active attention and responsibility. And every welcoming encounter differs from every other in the details of what attention unveils and what responsibility demands. Welcome is not a formulaic system into which we must fit ourselves. It is a way of living that, over time, comes to fit us, that we each make our own.

Over the years that the two of us have developed the concepts laid out in this book, we have each been learning, in our own particular ways, what it can mean to live the kind of life that an ethics of welcome calls for. As our commitment and understanding deepen, we see patterns of welcome (and unwelcome) everywhere. We find that we are increasingly aware of when we are and are not paying attention, breaking through stereotypes, imagining a story, imposing an agenda, letting someone come as they are—and increasingly aware that there remains so much more to do.

That is, these past several years have been for us an experience of letting this ethics of welcome make its home in us and of trying to live up to it. We now invite you to do the same. Live with it, practice it, make it your own. Let your experiences of being welcoming (and not) and of being welcomed (and not) interpret, embellish, and give further substance to the ideas in this book.

This is the dance we invited you to join in the closing words of our Introduction. The music is the embracing, multifaceted vision of a world in which human beings flourish, a world revealed and enabled by welcome. The steps are yours.

Dance with us toward a more welcoming world.

Note

1 Thomas Merton, *Conjectures of a Guilty Bystander* (Doubleday, New York, 1966), 153–4.

Epilogue

Further Steps

A week after learning that we had a book contract, one of us sat on the front porch of a neighbor's house in a small fishing town in the Canadian province of Nova Scotia. Talk turned to the book project, and the neighbor, Laura, after listening intently, said with some sadness that she does not feel welcomed in the community and, most acutely, in her church. She had "come from away," as the locals call it, seven years before, moving from a larger city in Ontario to settle in this town. She explained that people here are friendly to her and her husband but seem to think that is enough, and it isn't.

What would it take for her to feel welcomed? Laura thought for a while. Church members do know her and her husband's names but not much more about them. Then she clarified what appeared to bother her most: in the seven years she has been there, lifelong church members have never asked her to do anything. She felt that she had had to "force" herself on them eventually, volunteering to teach Sunday School and do other tasks. She wants instead to be asked to do things, to contribute to the community's efforts. Even though she is now involved in these endeavors, she is still never asked to do anything by anyone.

How does an ethics of welcome unpack this desire to be *asked* to give of one's time, to do tasks that might be considered chores or require sacrifices? The desire seems to involve something more and other than simply wanting one's talents to be acknowledged, to be recognized as someone who has much to offer (see Patterns 7 and 15). Perhaps it's the desire to feel that one now truly "belongs." Laura shared this as a story about welcome or, rather, the lack of it. Is there another pattern here? Very possibly so.

There are more patterns of welcome to be sorted through than we have assembled here. Everyone has stories that relate to the patterns within this book and to patterns that remain to be recognized and studied and placed within the language of welcome. They are personal and secondhand experiences; they happened recently and long ago; they arise in varied settings—churches, workplaces, parks, classrooms, family reunions. They may come from something we read or lived through or observed somewhere long ago, something that has stuck with us, though we are not sure why.

We invite readers to expand and enrich this ethics of welcome with your own stories and to recognize new patterns of welcome. That's what we've been doing for fifteen years, and we are keenly aware of how much more there is to understand and to tell.

Where might Laura's story fit among the patterns in this book—or where would a new pattern, fashioned around her story, belong? What about your story, your new pattern?

Appendix

To assist the continuation of this project, here is a summary list of the claims and imperatives that begin and end the patterns in the book. Where do your stories fit among them? What new patterns have you discovered?

Patterns of Welcome

Part I. What Welcome Is

1. Radical Openness

Welcome is a radical openness to the other person that both allows us to be moved and compels us to move in order to create, repair, and maintain the shared space necessary for responsible human relationships.

Open yourself to others as they are. Allow yourself to be moved by them.

2. Responding Rather Than Reacting

Welcome is not a reaction but a *response* to the particular person before us.

Learn to recognize reactions for what they are. Choose instead to respond.

3. Action

Welcome is openness and responsive action.

Move!—in response to internal stirrings engendered by another person *or* in order to be so affected by them. Act!—responsively and responsibly.

4. Step into the Room

Welcome is a physical act that overcomes the distance between persons.

Move closer. Enter the room, pull up a chair, write the note, make eye contact, nod to the stranger, return the phone call, make a video call. Take a step, physical or virtual, toward the other person.

5. Stay Awhile

Once one has moved toward the other person in welcome, it is not time for a hasty retreat. Welcome is a willingness to "stay in the room," to be present and share space, at least long enough to recognize the other person's uniqueness and our responsibilities to them.

Stay! Listen to the other person's story, their expressions of pain, sorrow, hope, joy. Hold their silence. Stay especially when a person is in need. Express your willingness to stay, if possible. Stay long enough to recognize the next step in welcome.

6. Invite the Other Person in

The space welcome creates is *shared* space in which each participant is willing to be open not only to receiving but also to offering some degree of self-revelation.

Pay attention to your boundaries; keep them from blocking your ability to be welcoming. As part of your openness to the other person, let them know you, at least a bit.

7. Everyone Is at Home

Welcome is a shared space where everyone is at home and has something equally valuable to offer.

Welcome makes possible balanced giving and receiving. As you welcome others, do not think of or present yourself as the one who gives or serves as host or sets the terms of the engagement.

8. Welcoming Ourselves

Welcome is owed to all, including ourselves.

Welcome yourself just as you welcome others.

Part II. Paying Attention

9. See a Human Being

First and always, you and I and they are human beings.

Recognize that the person we welcome is fully human. Look beyond the absence of familiar cues; examine and step around the presence of contrary biases.

10. See *This* Human Being

Sharing a common humanity does not mean that we are alike in all the ways that matter. Each person we welcome is unique, with their own particular way of being in the world.

Acknowledge the persons you welcome as unique individuals so that you may come to know them as they are and as they want to be known.

11. Who Is This Person *Right Now*?

Welcome requires paying attention to who people are now, in the moment of our encounter, whether they are a stranger or someone we've known well over a long time.

When encountering someone for the first time, pay attention to the cues that can help you see them as they are in that moment. When interacting with someone you know, draw on your well-established knowledge but also pay close attention to who they are right now.

12. Empathy Is Not Enough

There are perils in trying to know another person by imagining how they feel or experience life, even when we mean well. Welcome and empathy call for different strategies for knowing and connecting with another person.

Rely less on your imagination of what other persons might be experiencing. Instead, find out what their life is like from them or those close to them, if possible.

13. Everything about a Person Matters

Seeing the other person as they are, a distinctive and whole individual, is an act of respect and an essential component of welcome. It requires that we break through deeply ingrained tendencies to stereotype.

Step beyond the temptation to stereotype others. Reconsider them, again and again.

Part III. Things We Can Do

14. Practice, Practice, Practice

Becoming a welcoming person doesn't happen automatically, just because we wish it to be so. Rather, we have to practice welcoming behaviors and allow the practice itself, and what we learn from others' responses to us, to shape us into the welcoming persons we desire to be.

Practice all the possible ways of expressing your welcome to others. Practice and practice and practice.

15. Reconsider, Again and Again

There are many ways to reconsider the person we welcome, to break away from the generic categories we are tempted to assign.

Take another, more attentive and open look at the other person. Reconsider them with curiosity, generosity, and imagination.

16. Let People Tell You Who They Are

The best source for learning about the other person is that person.

Let the person you welcome tell you—by word, cry, gesture, demeanor—what you need to know in order to form a response that fits this unique person and this one of a kind encounter.

17. Pay Attention to Names

Names are our deepest, most fundamental identification of ourselves. Names require care; they require that we not be careless with them.

Practice getting others' names right.

18. Come as You Are

How we present ourselves and how we respond to others' reactions to our self-presentation can help or hinder the formation of welcoming relationships. It is possible to be true to ourselves and, at the same time, to be aware of how we present ourselves to others.

Be thoughtful about your self-presentation, anticipating and responding to others' reactions in ways that foster welcome while also remaining true to yourself.

19. Let Others Come as They Are

How others present themselves has an effect on whether and how we welcome them. Part of practicing welcome is paying attention to this influence, moving from reaction to response.

Be thoughtful about others' self-presentation. Be open to their choices and give them the benefit of the doubt.

20. Check Your Agenda

Welcome permits no hidden agendas.

Examine your agenda. Be sure that each purpose is compatible with welcome.

21. Worry Less about Being Manipulated

Excessive concern that we are being manipulated—and the injury to pride associated with it—can prevent us from engaging in welcoming behaviors.

Worry less about whether someone is trying to manipulate you. Learn to shrug a little more readily. Ask yourself what really matters here and now.

22. Be Open to Interruptions

Routine and habitual ways of doing and thinking can be highly useful as we go about our daily activities. But they can also make us less open to being interrupted by the persons in front of us, especially those who call for unexpected responses.

Look up. Listen up. Pick up the phone.

23. Put People before Principles

The principles by which we order our moral lives can only be comprehended by welcoming others.

Be loyal to your principles, in all their complexity and strength, by being open to learning from those whom you welcome what the rules mean in this moment and require in response.

24. Help Others Welcome You

We may, at times, encounter persons who appear not to welcome us in return. Although this can be a clear signal that no meaningful connection is possible—and should be respected as such—it may also be the case that, by our own welcoming approaches, we can help the other person welcome us.

In situations when the refusal of a welcome is not clear, if possible, take a moment of expectant silence or gentle exploration to see if you can help the other person welcome you.

Part IV. How Far Do We Have to Go?

25. Welcome Can Be Costly

The potential costs of welcoming another person can sometimes be too high for us to engage in welcoming actions. More often, we can responsibly balance our obligation to welcome and our obligation to care well for ourselves.

Be prepared for the risks involved in opening yourself to someone else. Only you can decide whether the risk is too much, whether the potential cost is more than you can bear.

26. Managing Aversions: No One Is Unworthy of Being Welcomed

Every person can be welcomed.

When welcoming someone is particularly difficult, or even seems impossible, remember that everyone deserves to be welcomed by someone. Ask, "Is it me? Why not me?"

27. Making Choices, Setting Limits

When the costs of welcoming another person are high—when what an ethics of welcome asks seems to be too much to expect of ourselves—we can make choices about our approaches and responses, setting limits as necessary while still maintaining a welcoming orientation.

Set limits as needed *within* welcome in open, responsive ways that are fitting for you and for the other person. Set limits *on* welcome only when absolutely necessary because of unacceptably high costs, and be willing to periodically reevaluate the scope of those limits. Always maintain a welcoming orientation.

28. Sharing the Responsibility

Responsibility to welcome others in the human community belongs to everyone and should be shared. Sharing the responsibility for welcome is essential for human flourishing.

Build nests. Allow and encourage others to join in your welcoming actions. See that those expected to be welcoming (all of us) are also experiencing welcome and the support it gives. Be aware of or ask for your own needed support.

29. A Fundamental View of the World

Wherever and whyever people gather, whether in the formal structures of an institution, by happenstance of geographical location, or out of a common interest or a shared goal, they take on group responsibilities to be welcoming.

Build welcoming communities at work, in your neighborhood, among people with whom you share particular interests. Invite others to join. Learn to spot when group practices, whether acts or omissions, contribute to unwelcoming environments. Work to change them.

Acknowledgments

This work has been one of the most fulfilling projects we have undertaken over our long careers, and we have worked every step of the way as partners and friends. We hardly know any longer who drafted what and who first came up with any particular idea. In the last several years, we often found ourselves at our favorite meeting spot, Cville Coffee, discussing the 15th or 100th iteration of a pattern, and one of us would say, "I really like how you phrased this," and the other would say, "Oh, you wrote that." So, first, we would like to acknowledge *each other* and the special time spent debating ideas, parsing words, questioning, praising, and supporting each other as we explored the depths of welcome and what it could mean for our lives and the lives of others.

Which leads us to another point: when you coauthor a work, there is the question of how to order the authors' names. But there truly is no traditionally understood "first author" of this book. We determined authorship order by flipping a coin.

There are many people to whom we owe our gratitude for contributions to this book. They include, of course, the authors of the many great works we have drawn from, from ancient writers like Aristotle and Sophocles to more modern thinkers such as Emmanuel Levinas and Margaret Urban Walker, plus historians, poets, advocates, and songwriters. We have endeavored, in our in-text citations and endnotes, to acknowledge our reliance on their work.

We owe a special debt of gratitude to our spouses for their wisdom, encouragement, engagement, patience, and unflagging support, as well as for their many helpful conversations about the book, its ideas, structure, and style.

Paul Shepherd, Lois' spouse, first suggested we write a book together after he read Margaret's *Attending Children* soon after Lois joined the faculty at the University of Virginia. He didn't know what subject the book should cover, but he was taken by Margaret's prose and thought the two of us shared a view of the world that could be explored and developed more deeply in book form. He also encouraged us to look at the structure and style of *A Pattern Language*.

Deborah Healey, Margaret's spouse, has been an enthusiastic cheerleader for this project from the moment of conception. Her certainty of both the importance of the topic and our ability to explain it in an accessible way was a firm anchor in rocky times. She offered insights from her career in medicine and her work, in retirement, as a lay minister that added depth and nuance to many facets of our topic, and her sharp, musical ear often helped us achieve the tone we were seeking.

We have gathered stories and illustrations, suggestions for further reading, and supportive and constructively critical comments from many students, colleagues, friends, family members, acquaintances, and audience members. There are so many that we are likely to forget to mention some, and we also do not know the names of them all. We are nevertheless grateful to every one of them, especially the countless medical and law students at the University of Virginia from whom we have learned so much. We would also like to offer our particular thanks for stories and bits of shared wisdom included in this book that came from the following individuals: Danny Becker, Roz Chast, Jim and Marcia Childress, Julia Connelly, Walt Davis, Peggy Galloway, Doris Greiner, Susan Hoffman, David Kangas, Joe Kovaz, Carolyn Lineberger, Bob MacCaughelty, Dea Mahanes, Ray Mohrmann, Larry Palmer, Jim and Peggy Plews-Ogan, Ben Sturgill, Julia Taylor, Erika Walker, and Linda Wielinga.

We received invaluable editorial assistance and reviews from Richard Brown, our editor at Bloomsbury/Rowman & Littlefield, from Paul Shepherd, and from helpful anonymous peer reviewers.

We thank the following groups and institutions, who invited presentations of aspects of this work (mostly given by Margaret), for the opportunity to speak, for audience members' insights and stories—some of which are included in the book—and for both welcoming and challenging us: Congregation Beth Israel, Charlottesville, Virginia; Deaconess Beth Israel Medical Center, Boston, Massachusetts; Loyola University and Loyola University Medical Center, Chicago, Illinois; Medicine and Ministry of the Whole Person Annual Meeting, Hendersonville, North Carolina; Mercy Medical Center, Baltimore, Maryland; National Association of Oncology Social Workers Annual Meeting,

Tampa, Florida; Peninsula Regional Medical Center and Salisbury University, Salisbury, Maryland; Providence Health & Services, Portland, Oregon; Sentara Center for Healthcare Ethics, Williamsburg, Virginia; Spectrum Hospital System, Grand Rapids, Michigan; Stephen Ministers of St. Paul's Memorial Church, Charlottesville, Virginia; UVA School of Nursing Compassionate Care Initiative, Charlottesville, Virginia; Wake Forest University School of Law, Winston-Salem, North Carolina. In addition, we thank the University of Virginia, its Schools of Medicine and Law, and the Center for Health Humanities and Ethics for their support over the years.

Finally, we are grateful to you, dear reader, for sharing in our quest for a more welcoming world.

Index

Note: Page numbers followed by 'n' indicates note numbers

Abse, Dannie   192–5, 218
acknowledgement   78
agenda(s)   153–8
Angelou, Maya   125–6
Annas, George   73 n.6
argument as dance   6
Aristotle   110–11
Arras, John   162 n.2
attention, paying attention   36, 55, 81, 116, 135–41, 199
aversions   199–208

Barnard, David   224
Belluck, Pam   176
bigotry   55, 69–71, 182–3, 192–5, 216–17, 225
boundaries   46–50
Bowlin, John R.   209 n.4

Carpenter, Mary Chapin   117
categorizing persons, *see* stereotypes
Cavell, Stanley   78
Chambliss, Daniel   164
Charon, Rita   123 n.3
Chast, Roz   41, 86
Chesterton, G. K.   47
children   68, 83–4, 113–14
Christakis, Nicholas   174–5
Churchill, Larry   121
communitarian ethics   71–2
compassion, *see* empathy
congruence, *see* integrity
costs of welcoming   185, 189–97, 211–19
Covid-19 pandemic   33–6, 61
Croce, Jim   135
curious, curiosity   119–20

Death of a Salesman (Miller)   199
disability   69, 89, 92–7
The Diving Bell and the Butterfly (Bauby)   32
Doerries, Bryan   38
dress   143–7

empathy   23, 32–3, 89–98
equal regard   137–8, 203, 230
ethics of care   71, 222

"faking it"   113
find something to like   121
fitting response (Niebuhr)   18
Fitzgerald, Faith   119–20

Gawande, Atul   86
gender   70–1, 131, 147, 149–50
A Gentleman in Moscow (Towles)   19, 77
gift   52–4

Haywood, Carlton   133 n.4, 152 n.1
home   51–9, 229
hospitality   46, 51, 56–8
human being   67–8, 72, 75, 199–206
human flourishing   7, 52, 110, 212, 217, 221

imagination   89–93, 98
imagine a different story   122–3
institutions/institutional   3, 222, 231–2, 236
integrity   23, 26–7, 104, 111, 116
intention, intentional   12–15, 110, 155–6
interruption   30 n.4, 163–9, 184

justice   110–11, 183–4

Kangas, David   26
Kant, Immanuel   78
Kendi, Ibram X.   70
Kittay, Eva Feder   222

Lennon, John   166
Levinas, Emmanuel   3, 26, 30 n.4, 99 n.10, 115–16
limits   48–9, 161, 167, 211–19
listen, listening   125–32
liveable, liveability   5, 229–30
Longmore, Paul   94, 97
love   2, 23, 78, 240

manipulation, manipulative behavior   157–62
Mead, Rebecca   176
Merton, Thomas   239
Metaphors We Live By (Lakoff and Johnson)   6
Miller, Paul Steven   92
Miller, Richard   78
misericordia   13–14, 28
Moor, Ben   34–5
moving, movement   11–15, 23–30, 32, 36
Munson, Ronald   208 n.2
murderer(s)   3, 204–6

names, attention to   72, 135–41
names, misuse of   139–41
nested welcome   222–6, 234
Niebuhr, H. Richard   4, 18
non-linearity   6, 28
Nussbaum, Martha   48, 92

Ogletree, Thomas   46, 57
Opatrny, Lucie   52
openness   11–15, 29, 62

Palmer, Larry   75–6
A Pattern Language (Alexander, et al.)   5, 229
patterns   3, 5–6
persons   67–9, 103–4
perspective   2, 3, 219

phone call, ringing telephone   26, 168
"political correctness"   132
practice   48–9, 103, 109–18, 234
prejudice, prejudgments   183–4
principle(s)   171–8, 202–3
proximity   31–42, 204

racism, *see* bigotry
react, reactions   17–21, 144, 147–50, 184–5
recognition of humanness   67–79, 137
reconsider, reconsideration   103, 119–23
Regeneration (Barker)   46
religion, religious symbols   2–3, 146–7
respect   78, 137–8, 176–8, 184–5
response, responsive, responsibility   1–2, 17–22, 26, 30, 221–38
risks of welcoming   185, 189–97, 211, 217
role(s)   1, 27, 168–9
routinization   164
Runkel, Hal   174
rupture   116, 165

Schenck, David   121
self-presentation   143–52
sex offender(s)   206–7
sexism, *see* bigotry
shared space   11, 45–58
Shepherd, Paul   32
stereotypes, stereotyping   77, 101–5, 119–22
Stevenson, Bryan   204

Taylor, Julia   130
theme, thematizing   96
tolerance   200
Towles, Amor   19, 77
"truth dump"   174–5
truth-telling   171–8
typing persons, *see* stereotypes

United States Supreme Court   25–9

Venn diagram   58, 182
virtue   2, 14, 110, 115, 217

Walker, Margaret Urban 4, 227 n.4
Washington, Harriet 70
welcome
    action/movement 15, 23–30
    character trait, virtue, habit 2, 14, 110, 115, 217
    desire 12, 31, 55–6, 115
    etymology 12
    first work 2
    hospitality, distinction from 56–8
    mutual (ideal) 52–7, 181
    nested 222–6, 234
    not a gift 52–4
    not an expression of power 54–6
    obligation 2, 15, 189, 231–2
    of others as they are 1, 13, 41, 81, 149–52
    overcoming distance 28, 31–6
    of persons 40
    perspective(s) 2, 65–105
    policies 231–7
    practice(s) 107–86
    primary 2, 219, 232
    response, responsibility 17–22
    shared space 45–58
    welcoming orientation 12, 194, 205, 211–19
    welcoming ourselves 61–4, 196, 208
    willkommen 12
welcome mat 211–12, 216–17
White supremacy, *see* bigotry
wholeness, whole persons 32–3, 62–3, 103–5, 204
words in pocket 113, 164

"yes, and" 125–6, 160–1

Zoloth, Laurie 30 n.4, 168

Index of Stories

Alzheimer's Disease patients   176
"Australian angels", *see* Don and Moya Ritchie

baby in PICU   67
bearing, *see* Vivian Bearing
Black men in church, *see* Larry Palmer
Bouvia, *see* Elizabeth Bouvia
buttons and lanyards   143

Carolyn, Lois' mother   109–10
"Case History" poem   192
child with cystic fibrosis, *see* Jake and his prognosis
children feeling unwelcomed   83–4
chocolate ice cream and football, *see* Dr. Block's father
community members of the research ethics board   233–4
Cory, *see* children feeling unwelcomed
Count Rostov   19, 77, 103
Covid-19 patients   34–5

DeShaney, *see* Joshua DeShaney
Don and Moya Ritchie   11, 23, 29, 33, 112, 189
Dr. Block's father   86
Dr. Wilson, *see* Ms. Smythe and Dr. Wilson
Dwyer, *see* Rob Dwyer

Elizabeth Bouvia   94–5, 192
empathic wallpaper   46

Golden Gate Bridge, *see* Kevin Hines
Greek tragedy, *see* Philoctetes

heart transplant patient, *see* Rob Dwyer

Jacqueline Wilson, *see* Ms. Smythe and Dr. Wilson

Jake and his prognosis   171, 175–6
Jean Smythe, *see* Ms. Smythe and Dr. Wilson
John Rembert   17–18
Joshua DeShaney   25
JR, *see* John Rembert

Kevin Hines   81–2, 164

Larry Palmer   75–6
lawyer interrupted by client   165–6
lay minister and her garden   213–14
legislators in PICU, *see* baby in PICU
Lois' mother, *see* Carolyn

man on bridge, *see* Kevin Hines
Mara's grandmother   85
Margaret being called "sir"   61–2
Margaret in the ER   136–7
Marion and Dr. Achebe   127
Mark Horowitz   24
medical case study, *see* John Rembert
medical ethicist and heart transplant patient, *see* Rob Dwyer
medical student and honey farmer   45
medical student who walks past the door   23, 26–9
Michael, *see* children feeling unwelcomed
Moor, Ben, *see* Covid-19 patients
Ms. B   93–4
Ms. Smythe and Dr. Wilson   182–3, 194, 211, 215–16, 224–5

Neoptolemus, *see* Philoctetes
nurse with obese patient   101

organ procurement organization (OPO) in ICU   153, 234–5

patient who warmed doctor's hands   51–2
Philoctetes   37–8

Index of Stories

rehabilitation specialist   89
removing life support, court cases, *see* Elizabeth Bouvia, Ms. B
resident who sits down with patient, *see* Mark Horowitz
Ritchies, *see* Don and Moya Ritchie
Rob Dwyer   199–200
Roz Chast and her mother   41, 86
Ruth, Mickey, and Mary   31–2, 39–40

Samaritan   13
Sarah Philips   139, 141
school and student with epilepsy   222–3
sickle cell disease patients   128, 151
Social Security, *see* lawyer interrupted
store clerk in costume   152
stroke patient, *see* Sarah Philips
student asking for paper extension, *see* Vivian Bearing
Supreme Court case, *see* Joshua DeShaney

terminally ill or dying patients, *see* COVID-19 patients, Elizabeth Bouvia, Mara's grandmother, Mark Horowitz, medical student who walks past the door, Ms. B, Roz Chast and her mother, Ruth, Mickey, and Mary
Titanic survivor   119–20
transgendered patient and doctor's reaction   149
"trouble thinking", *see* Alzheimer's Disease patients
TSA agent   163
tuberculosis patient wandering around the hospital   158

university health system's response to bigotry   216, 225

Vivian Bearing   157

W;t (Edson)   157
welcome mat   211–12, 216–17
White supremacist activities   216, 237

"You're Black!", *see* Ms. Smythe and Dr. Wilson